# Current Clinical Practice

D0985521

**Series Editor**
Neil S. Skolnik
Temple University, School of Medicine, Abington Memorial Hospital,
Abington, PA, USA

For further volumes:
http://www.springer.com/series/7633

Steven Hollenberg · Stephen Heitner

# Cardiology in Family Practice

A Practical Guide

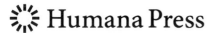 Humana Press

Steven Hollenberg
Cooper University Hospital
Camden, NJ, USA
Hollenbergsteven@cooperhealth.edu

Stephen Heitner
Robert Wood Johnson Medical School
University of Medicine and Dentistry
of Section of Cardiology
Cooper University Hospital
Camden, NJ, USA

ISBN 978-1-61779-384-4        e-ISBN 978-1-61779-385-1
DOI 10.1007/978-1-61779-385-1
Springer New York Dordrecht Heidelberg London

Library of Congress Control Number: 2011936745

Humana Press is part of Springer Science+Business Media (www.springer.com)

# Preface

Cardiovascular disease is an enormous problem in industrialized nations. Despite a declining incidence, an estimated 70 million Americans have some form of cardio-vascular disease, which takes more than 830,000 lives and prompts 6,200,000 hospital admissions each year. Given the aging of the population and the challenges in risk factor management, these numbers are more likely to increase than decrease. In fact, better management of acute phases has led to an increased number of patients with chronic manifestations of cardiovascular disease.

The response has been a prodigious effort on all fronts. Classic cardiovascular research encompasses physiology and pharmacology, but has now grown to include genetics, genomics, epidemiology, molecular biology, developmental biology, and biophysics, bioengineering, and information technology, all of which are taking advantage of an impressive and ever-increasing set of sophisticated investigational tools. Old paradigms are under constant assault from a barrage of new information. Clinical research has developed just as quickly, generating a voluminous body of trial data that seems to grow exponentially.

All of this poses its own set of problems for practitioners, in particular those without subspecialty training in cardiovascular disease. The rate of advance of clinical cardiology continues to accelerate, with new pathophysiologic models, new imaging technologies, and new therapies. Meanwhile, the volume of cardiac patients, particularly in the hospital setting, is increasing.

With all of this in mind, we offer up this short volume, neither exhaustive nor all-encompassing, but designed to be clear and concise. We hope to promote under-standing of basic mechanisms underlying disease states, since these provide the rationales for treatment strategies. The emphasis, however, is on delineating practical techniques for evaluation and treatment of patients with cardiovascular problems. Along the same lines, references are not meant to be comprehensive but to point the reader to the most useful sources of additional information. Our goal is to provide a fast and effective way for practitioners to identify important concepts and information that they can use to deliver more effective patient care.

Camden, NJ                                                    Steven Hollenberg
Camden, NJ                                                     Stephen Heitner

# Series Editor's Introduction

Family doctors see patients with cardiac risk factors and cardiac disease every single day, and each day they make decisions about the medical care of those patients. Over the last 20 years, there has been an explosion of knowledge and therapeutic choices for caring for patients with cardiac risk factors and disease. Heart disease accounts for 700,000 deaths per year in the United States, accounting for 28% of all annual deaths in the country [1]. In 2004, family doctors prescribed 29% of all cardiovascular drugs prescribed nationwide during approximately 70 million office visits [2].

*Cardiology in Family Practice: A Practical Guide*, second edition, by Drs. Steven Hollenberg and Stephen Heitner, is an erudite book that is unique for its short length combined with its breadth, covering the range of cardiovascular risk factors and diseases that primary care physicians encounter in both inpatient and outpatient settings. The authors provide readers with information to competently care for patients and make clear diagnostic and therapeutic choices based on the best evidence currently available. They do this with a clarity of voice that is unusual in medical writing. *Cardiology in Family Practice* should be useful to all physicians in primary care who are looking to update their knowledge of cardiac disease, and who would like a concise, relevant textbook to read and refer to on their shelves.

Neil S. Skolnik, MD

# References

1. US National Center for Health Statistics. Cause of Death. http://www.cdc.gov/nchs/data/dvs/LCWK1_2002.pdf. Accessed 13 September 2005.
2. US Department of Health and Human Services, Public Health Service, Centers for Disease Control and Prevention, National Care for Health Statistics, 2002 data. Public Use data file. http://www.aafp.org/x796.xml. Accessed 13 September 2005.

# Contents

# Chapter 1
# Stable Angina

## Definition and Pathophysiology

Myocardial ischemia results from an imbalance of oxygen supply and oxygen demand. Traditionally, myocardial ischemia has been differentiated in terms of the acuity and stability of the symptoms. Typical angina is exertional, and is relieved promptly by rest or nitroglycerin. Stable angina occurs reproducibly with a similar level of exertion, in a pattern that is unchanged over the last 6 months. In 2006, despite therapeutic advances, 9.8 million patients had angina in the United States [1]. New, worsening, or rest symptoms, and chest pain associated with elevated cardiac enzymes, fall under the category of the acute coronary syndromes (unstable angina, ST- and non-ST-segment elevation myocardial infarction) and is discussed in the appropriate chapter.

## *Pathophysiology*

The heart is an aerobic organ with only a limited capacity for anaerobic glycolysis. It makes use of oxygen avidly and efficiently, extracting 70–80% of the oxygen from coronary arterial blood [2]. Because the heart extracts oxygen nearly maximally and independent of demand, any increase in demand must be met by a commensurate increase in coronary blood flow. The myocardial requirement for oxygen, and hence for oxygenated blood, is affected by three major variables: heart rate, myocardial wall stress, and contractility. Myocardial wall stress is a function of the cavity radius, the myocardial wall thickness, and the intraventricular pressure which is highly dependent on ventricular afterload (see Fig. 1.1).

Coronary blood flow depends on coronary perfusion pressure and filling time. Since coronary perfusion occurs primarily during diastole, the perfusion pressure is the difference between diastolic pressures in the aorta and left ventricular cavity. Filling time is directly related to heart rate.

S. Hollenberg and S. Heitner, *Cardiology in Family Practice: A Practical Guide*,
Current Clinical Practice 1, DOI 10.1007/978-1-61779-385-1_1,
© Springer Science+Business Media, LLC 2012

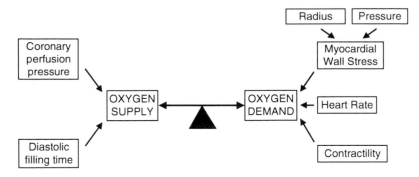

**Fig. 1.1** Determinants of myocardial oxygen supply and demand

Myocardial ischemia develops in the setting of a flow-limiting coronary artery obstruction that limits blood supply. The pathophysiology of unstable coronary syndromes and myocardial infarction (MI) usually involves dynamic, partial or complete occlusion of an epicardial coronary artery because of acute intracoronary thrombus formation [3]. This is described in the chapter on acute coronary syndromes.

A number of factors can increase myocardial oxygen demand, including tachycardia, hypertension, and increased catecholamines resulting from stress. Similarly, many factors could contribute to limitation of oxygen supply, particularly in the setting of hemodynamic instability. These factors include hypotension, decreasing coronary perfusion pressure, and tachycardia, limiting diastolic filling time. In addition, anemia and hypoxemia can limit the amount of oxygen delivered to the heart. Coronary vasospasm may also play a role in some patients. Elevation of left ventricular pressures, as seen in left-sided heart failure, can increase both demand (elevated afterload) and reduce coronary perfusion pressure.

## Diagnosis

### Signs and Symptoms

Heberden provided the first documentation of angina in 1768 – a painful sensation in the breast accompanied by a strangling sensation, anxiety, and occasional radiation of pain to the left arm. He also observed an association with exertion and relief with rest [4]. His description has remained accurate for almost three and a half centuries.

Angina most commonly manifests as a constant substernal tightness, pressure, or ache. The discomfort may radiate to the throat and jaw or to the left shoulder and left arm. This is often accompanied by acute onset of dyspnea and diaphoresis. The sensation may occasionally be right-sided, interscapular, or perceived in the epigastrium. While the history is vital when considering angina, chest pain that is myocardial in origin is notoriously heterogeneous, and a high level of suspicion should be maintained in all patients presenting with chest discomfort [5]. Descriptions that fit with Heberden's original syndrome are generally referred to as typical chest pain, whereas those with alternate or different features are referred to as atypical chest pain. A more contemporary classification into typical, atypical, and noncardiac chest pain is shown in Table 1.1 [6]. The severity of anginal symptoms can be rated from Class I to IV using the Canadian Cardiovascular Society classification (see Table 1.2).

| Table 1.1 Diamond classification of angina | Substernal chest discomfort<br>Exacerbated with exercise or emotional stress<br>Relieved by rest of nitroglycerin<br>Typical angina: All three features present<br>Atypical angina: One or two features present<br>Non-cardiac: No features present |
|---|---|
| | Adapted from Diamond [6] |

| Table 1.2 Canadian Cardiovascular Society Classification of Angina | | |
|---|---|---|
| | Class I | Symptoms only with strenuous activity |
| | Class II | Slight limitation in ordinary physical activity |
| | Class III | Marked limitation in ordinary physical activity |
| | Class IV | Symptoms with any activity or at rest |

The physical examination is generally insensitive and nonspecific, especially in patients with multiple comorbidities. Elevated jugular veins signal elevated right ventricular pressures, and pulmonary crackles (in the absence of pulmonary disease) indicate elevated left ventricular filling pressures. During the ischemic episode, auscultation of the precordium may reveal the presence of a fourth heart sound, indicative of a noncompliant left ventricle. In the presence of left ventricular systolic dysfunction, a third heart sound may be present. A holosystolic murmur of mitral regurgitation may result from papillary muscle ischemia, leading to functional mitral regurgitation.

## The Electrocardiogram

The electrocardiographic (ECG) abnormalities in myocardial ischemia vary widely and depend in large part on the extent and nature of coronary stenosis, the presence of prior myocardial infarction, whether there is preexisting conduction disease, and the extent of collateral blood flow to ischemic zones. Importantly, while the specificity of ECG abnormalities is relatively low for the confirmation of coronary disease, the presence of baseline abnormalities (especially left bundle branch block and Q-waves) is frequently associated with coronary disease. A detailed discussion of ECG interpretation is beyond the scope of this chapter.

The most prominent ECG changes with ischemia occur in the ST segment, which is normally isoelectric, since the cells have the same membrane potential during repolarization. Cellular ischemia lowers the resting potential and thus creates a voltage gradient between normal and ischemic areas, which shifts the ST segment.

In transmural ischemia, the ST-segment is shifted toward the epicardial layers, producing ST elevation (also known as "injury current"). With sub-endocardial ischemia, the ST segment is shifted toward the endocardium layers, producing ST depression. Classic angina produces ST depression.

The pattern of ECG changes may give a guide to the area and extent of infarction. The number of leads involved broadly reflects the extent of myocardium involved. Although localization of the area of ischemia is more accurate when the ST segments are elevated than when they are depressed, the general pattern is similar. Anterior ischemia is manifest in leads $V_1$–$V_4$, inferior ischemia in leads II, III, and aVF, and lateral ischemia in leads I, aVL, $V_5$, and $V_6$.

The ECG diagnosis of ischemia can be difficult in the presence of conduction abnormalities, especially with preexisting left bundle branch block. ST-depression can also be caused by medications (digitalis in particular), electrolyte disorders (frequently with hypokalemia), cardiomyopathies, myocarditis, supraventricular tachycardias, and cerebrovascular events. Left ventricular hypertrophy may also result in ST-depression – the so-called "strain" pattern.

## Differential Diagnosis

The differential diagnosis of chest discomfort is broad and includes gastrointestinal, pulmonary, musculoskeletal, and neurologic causes, which can sometimes be difficult to distinguish from cardiac symptoms, since the heart shares some sensory innervation with other thoracic organs. Pericarditis can present like ischemia, although the pain of pericarditis is more commonly sharp and pleuritic, and may be positional. Prominent gastrointestinal causes of chest pain include esophageal disorders such as reflux, spasm, other motility disorders, and esophageal rupture, peptic ulcer disease, cholecystitis, and pancreatitis [5, 7].

## Stress Testing

Patients with an intermediate probability of obstructive coronary artery disease (CAD) should be considered for stress testing to help with establishing a diagnosis. In patients with established CAD, stress testing provides a valuable means of prognostication and can aid in optimal decision-making. Of the testing modalities, symptom-limited exercise is preferred unless contraindicated (critical aortic stenosis), or if pharmacological testing is desirable because of ECG indications (preexisting left bundle branch block, ST-segment depression $\geq 1$ mm, ventricular paced rhythm, or

Wolff–Parkinson–White syndrome). The addition of imaging, either via nuclear tracer or echocardiography, improves sensitivity and specificity of the stress test, especially in the setting of an abnormal baseline ECG. Imaging also allows for anatomical localization of perfusion deficits in many instances. In conjunction with exercise, either echocardiographic images (looking for inducible wall motion abnormalities) or nuclear perfusion tracers (looking for relative perfusion defects) can be used to create both a physiologic and anatomic assessment, and is invaluable in formulating a prognosis, Should pharmacologic testing be necessary, either vasodilator (adenosine, regadenason, or dipyridamole) nuclear or chronotropic (dobutamine) agents can be used with either nuclear or echocardiographic imaging. The appropriateness criteria for each of these modalities have been published by the respective societies [8, 9].

## Treatment

The management of stable CAD is twofold: symptom control and prevention of cardiovascular events. Bearing in mind that myocardial ischemia results from an imbalance of myocardial oxygen supply and demand, patients may often be successfully treated simply by the removal of provocative stimuli that result in increased myocardial oxygen demand or decreased oxygen delivery. For example, correction of hypoxia, anemia, hypovolemia, tachycardia, or hypertension, may be sufficient to control anginal episodes.

Treatment of stable angina entails a combination of therapeutic interventions aimed at symptom relief as well as lifestyle modifications designed to minimize the potential complications. The mnemonic *ABCDE* combines the two conceptually, serving to emphasize the point that acute interventions are only the prelude to secondary prevention (chronic angina guidelines).

*A*spirin/Antiplatelets
*A*ntianginals
*B*eta blockers
*B*lood pressure control
*C*holesterol reduction
*C*igarettes: smoking cessation program
*D*ietary modification
*D*iabetes management
*E*ducation
*E*xercise

### *Aspirin*

Aspirin is the best known and the most widely used of all the antiplatelet agents because of low cost and relatively low toxicity. Use of salicylates to treat coronary artery disease in the United States was first reported in 1953 [10]. Aspirin inhibits the production of thromboxane $A_2$ by irreversibly acetylating the serine residue of the enzyme prostaglandin H2 synthetase.

Reduction of death or nonfatal myocardial infarction in patients with unstable angina and non-ST elevation myocardial infarction has been well established in several large randomized clinical trials [11, 12]. In addition to its use in acute clinical settings, aspirin has also been shown to be beneficial in preventing cardiovascular events when administered as secondary prevention in patients after acute myocardial infarction and as primary prevention in subjects with no prior history of vascular disease [13].

The most widely used and effective dose of aspirin in cardiovascular disease is between 81 and 325 mg daily. Apart from the fact that aspirin blocks thromboxane preferentially to prostacyclin at low doses and thus has a more profound antiplatelet effect, high-dose aspirin has been found to be as effective as low-dose aspirin in prevention of cardiovascular death, myocardial infarction, and stroke [14], which may suggest that besides its antiplatelet effects, anti-inflammatory effects of aspirin play a role as well [15]. Once begun, aspirin should probably be continued indefinitely. Toxicity with aspirin is mostly gastrointestinal; enteric-coated preparations may minimize these side effects.

Some data support clopidogrel use in patients at risk of developing cardiovascular complications [16], but its use in isolation as a part of therapy in chronic stable angina has not been well characterized and it should only be considered when aspirin is contraindicated (e.g. aspirin allergy), or if there is a separate indication for its use (e.g. coronary stent deployment within the last year, recent myocardial infarction, or stroke).

## Antianginals: Nitrates

Nitroglycerin is a mainstay of therapy for angina because of its efficacy and rapid onset of action. The most important antianginal effect of nitroglycerin is the preferential dilation of venous capacitance vessels, decreasing venous return. A reduction in myocardial oxygen demand and consumption results from the reduction of LV volume and arterial pressure primarily due to reduced preload [17]. At higher doses, in some patients, nitroglycerin relaxes arterial smooth muscle as well, causing a modest decrease in afterload, which contributes to a decrement in wall stress [17]. In addition, nitroglycerin can dilate epicardial coronary arteries as well as redistribute coronary blood flow to ischemic regions by dilating collateral vessels. Nitroglycerin has also been shown to have antithrombotic and antiplatelet effects [18].

Nitroglycerin is useful in treating acute angina episodes, with successive sublingual administration of 0.4 mg often providing rapid resolution of symptoms. Short-acting nitrates can also be used pre-emptively a few minutes prior to exertion. Topical or longer acting oral nitrates may be used in conjunction with ß-blockers and calcium channel antagonists and have been shown to be effective as a means to decreasing the frequency of angina [19].

Because of its hemodynamic actions, systemic blood pressure may fall after nitroglycerin administration, and patients should be warned about potential postural hypotension and falls. Should symptomatic hypotension occur, it can be effectively treated by placing the patient in the Trendelenburg position or by giving intravenous saline boluses. Hypotension is exacerbated in the event of concomitant phosphodi-esterase inhibitor use (such as sildenafil), and concurrent use is contraindicated. The most frequent side effect of nitrates is headache. Tolerance usually develops over time and patients should be encouraged to persist with the drug until this occurs. Unfortunately, tolerance to the beneficial effects of nitrates also develops, and periods of drug cessation and reintroduction (drug holidays) can be used as a means to resensitize a patient to the antianginal effects.

## Antianginals: β-Blockers

The rationale for administration of ß-blockers during ischemic episodes derives from their negative chronotropic and negative inotropic properties. Heart rate and contractility are two of the three major determinants of myocardial oxygen consumption. By altering these variables, myocardial ischemia, through decreasing oxygen demand, can be attenuated significantly [20]. These agents are particularly effective in patients with angina who remain tachycardic or hypertensive (or both) and in patients with supraventricular tachycardia complicating myocardial ischemia. Rapid control can be achieved by intravenous administration of metoprolol, a $ß_1$-selective blocker, in 5 mg increments every 5 min up to 15 mg. Thereafter, 25–50 mg every 6 h can be given orally. ß-Blockers should be used with caution in patients with marginal blood pressure, preexisting bradycardia, AV nodal conduction disturbances, and evidence for left ventricular failure, as well as those with bronchial hyper-reactivity. Diabetes is not a contraindication to ß-blocker therapy, and in fact the absolute risk reduction may be greater in these patients since they are at higher cardiovascular risk.

## Antianginals: Calcium Channel Blockers

Non-dihydropyridine calcium channel blockers (verapamil and diltiazem) also have negative chronotropic and inotropic effects, and can be used to control myocardial oxygen demand in patients with ischemia. Both can be given as intravenous boluses, starting with low doses (diltiazem 10–20 mg, verapamil 2.5 mg), and can then be infused continuously.

Calcium channel blockers are particularly useful in the setting of coronary vasospasm, because they cause direct dilation of coronary vascular smooth muscle. Vasospasm can produce variant angina in patients with mild or no coronary artery disease (Prinzmetal's angina), or aggravate ischemia in patients with atherosclerotic coronary stenoses that are subcritical but serve as sites of vasospasm, possibly as a consequence of abnormalities of the underlying smooth muscle or derangements in endothelial physiology [21]. The illicit use of cocaine is increasingly being recognized as a cause of coronary vasospasm leading to angina and myocardial ischemia. Coronary vasospasm usually presents with ST elevation associated with chest pain, and can be difficult to differentiate from vessel closure due to coronary thrombosis. Consideration of the clinical setting, rapid fluctuation of ST segments, and prompt resolution with nitrates can provide useful clues. Variant angina attributable to vasospasm responds well to treatment with calcium channel blockers.

Short-acting dihydropyridine calcium blockers, however, have been associated with increased cardiovascular risk with long-term use, and should in general be avoided. A similar risk has not been shown, however, for extended release preparations [22].

## Antianginals: Ranolazine

Ranolazine is a novel antianginal agent that has recently been approved by the FDA for use in conjunction with other antianginal drugs. Its mechanism of action is through alteration of sodium-dependent calcium release in cardiomyocytes. Ranolazine was recently shown to be superior to placebo at decreasing anginal episode frequency and severity, as well as increasing exercise capacity [23].

## Blood Pressure Control

Antihypertensive therapy has been shown to reduce the incidence of myocardial infarction by 20–25%, heart failure by more than 50%, and stroke by 35–40% [24]. Clearly, hypertensive control is of paramount importance in both the acute and chronic management of angina. In patients with coronary artery disease, the goal blood pressure is less than 130/80 mmHg [25, 26]. A complete description of the topic can be found in the Hypertension chapter in this book.

## Angiotensin-Converting Enzyme Inhibitors

Angiotensin-converting enzyme (ACE) generates angiotensin II from angiotensin I as well as catalyzing the breakdown of bradykinin. Consequently, ACE inhibitors decrease circulating angiotensin II levels and increase levels of bradykinin, which in turn stimulates production of nitric oxide by endothelial nitric oxide synthase. In the vasculature, ACE inhibition promotes vasodilation, and tends to inhibit smooth muscle proliferation, platelet aggregation, and thrombosis.

The major hemodynamic effect of ACE inhibition is afterload reduction, which is most important as an influence on myocardial oxygen demand in patients with impaired left ventricular function. The HOPE trial randomized 9,297 patients with documented vascular disease or those at high risk for atherosclerosis (diabetes plus at least one other risk factor) in the absence of heart failure to treatment with the tissue-selective ACE inhibitor ramipril (target dose 10 mg/day) or placebo and showed a 22% reduction in the combined endpoint of cardiovascular death, myocardial infarction (MI), and stroke [27]. Cardiovascular risk reduction in patients with stable angina was also found using perindopril in the EUROPA trial [28]. More recently, the PEACE trial, which compared trandolapril to placebo in 8,290 patients with stable coronary artery disease, found no significant difference in death, myocardial infarction, or need for revascularization [29]. The reason for these differences remains unclear; lipid control was better in the PEACE trial, but differences in the drugs cannot be excluded.

On the basis of these data, the most recent ACC/AHA guidelines recommend the use of ACE inhibitors in patients with stable angina and moderate to severe LV dysfunction, and in patients with diabetes mellitus. ACE inhibitors can be considered in patients with mild or normal left ventricular systolic dysfunction. Angiotensin receptor blockers (ARBs) can be substituted for ACE inhibitors in patients who are unable to tolerate ACE inhibitors. ACE inhibitors and ARBs are contraindicated in patients with severe renal insufficiency not on dialysis [30, 31].


## Cholesterol Reduction

There is extensive epidemiologic, laboratory, and clinical evidence linking cholesterol and coronary artery disease. Total cholesterol level has been linked to the development of CAD events with a continuous and graded relation [30]. Most of this risk is due to LDL cholesterol. A number of large primary and secondary prevention trials have shown that LDL cholesterol lowering is associated with a reduced risk of coronary disease events. Earlier lipid-lowering trials used bile-acid sequestrants (cholestyramine), fibric acid derivatives (gemfibrozil and clofibrate), or niacin, in addition to diet. The reduction in total cholesterol in these early trials was 6–15% and was accompanied by a consistent trend toward a reduction in fatal and nonfatal coronary events [31].

More impressive results have been achieved using HMG-CoA reductase inhibitors (statins). Statins have been demonstrated to decrease the rate of adverse ischemic events in patients with documented CAD in the 4S trial [32], as well as in the CARE study [33] and the LIPID trial [34]. On the basis of these trials, the last National Cholesterol Education Program (NCEP) guidelines proposed an LDL cholesterol level less than 130 mg/dL as a treatment goal [35], but an update based on more recent data recommended an even lower LDL target of less than 100 mg/dL [36]. Maximum benefit may require management of other lipid abnormalities (elevated triglycerides, low HDL cholesterol) and treatment of other atherogenic risk factors.

Since the publication of those guidelines, however, results of several trials have emerged. The PROVE-IT trial randomized 4,162 patients with acute coronary syndromes to pravastatin (40 mg daily, standard therapy) 80 mg of atorvastatin daily (80 mg, intensive therapy). LDL cholesterol was 125 mg/dL at baseline, and was lowered more in the intensive therapy group (to 62 mg/dL) than in the standard therapy group (95 mg/dL). This reduction was associated with a significant reduction in primary end point (a composite of death, myocardial infarction, unstable angina, revascularization, and stroke), from 26.3 to 22.4%, $p=0.005$ [37]. The REVERSAL trial showed that intensive lipid-lowering treatment with atorvastatin, which lowered LDL cholesterol from 150 to 79 mg/dL reduced progression of coronary atherosclerosis, as assessed by intracoronary ultrasound, compared with a moderate regimen that lowered LDL to 110 mg/dL [38]. These trials suggest that such patients benefit from early and continued lowering of LDL cholesterol to levels substantially below current target levels. Recent additions to the practice guidelines for chronic angina include consideration of adding plant stanol/sterols (2 g/day) and/or viscous fiber (greater than 10 g/day) to further lower LDL-C [39]. A complete discussion of the role of dyslipidemia in coronary artery disease, as well as up-to-date management strategies is provided in Chap. 9.

## Cigarette Smoking

Cigarette smoking is the most important alterable risk factor contributing to premature morbidity and mortality in the United States. Smoking acts synergistically with other risk factors, and the risk is strongly dose-related. As many as 30% of all coronary heart disease deaths in the United States each year are directly attributable to cigarette smoking. Smoking also doubles the risk of ischemic stroke.

Smoking cessation decreases the risk of coronary morbidity and mortality as well as stroke, with a diminution of risk that starts very soon after quitting, but also progresses over time. Benefits can, however, be obtained from smoking cessation even after many years of smoking and after presentation of smoking related disease. In fact, development of clinical illness often represents a "teachable moment" during which patients are highly motivated to change their lifestyle. The provision of a multicomponent smoking cessation program, with or without pharmacotherapy, is associated with a 50% long-term (more than 1 year) smoking cessation rate in patients who have been hospitalized with a coronary event, and telephone-based counseling has the potential to increase this to 70% [40].

There is overwhelming evidence demonstrating both the cardiovascular hazards of smoking and the prompt benefit that occurs with smoking cessation. The provision of advice alone significantly increases the smoking cessation rate, and even minimal counseling yields further benefit. Intervention with patients who have already suffered a cardiac event yields particularly striking benefits. The smoking status of all patients should be assessed and appropriate intervention should be offered to those who smoke [39].

## Diet

Dietary management is of clear importance for the management of coronary heart disease. On a population level, limitation of dietary saturated fat to <10% of energy and cholesterol to <300 mg/day, but specific recommendations for individuals should be based on cholesterol and lipoprotein levels and the presence of diabetes and other risk factors. Studies support a major benefit on blood pressure of consuming vegetables, fruits, and low-fat dairy products, as well as limiting salt intake (<6 g/day) and alcohol (no more than two drinks per day for men and one for women) and maintaining a healthy body weight. Consumption of at least two fish servings per week is now recommended on the basis of evidence that consumption of omega-3 fatty acids confers cardiovascular benefits [41].

Obesity is being increasingly recognized as an important risk factor for coronary artery disease and thus an important target for preventive strategies. Being overweight is associated with an increased incidence and prevalence of hypertension and diabetes before and during adulthood as well as with the later development of cardiovascular disease in adults. A constellation of risk factors known as the metabolic syndrome (abdominal obesity, high triglycerides and low HDL, hypertension, and insulin resistance) confers a particularly high risk of cardiac disease and complications. When body mass index (BMI) is excessive, caloric intake should be less than energy expended in physical activity to reduce BMI. In general, relative caloric restriction sufficient to produce weight reductions between 5 and 10% can reduce the risk factors for heart disease and stroke. Weight loss programs that result in a slow but steady weight reduction (1–2 lb per week for up to 6 months) appear to be at least as efficacious as diets with more rapid initial weight loss over the long term and may be more effective in promoting the behavioral changes needed to maintain weight loss [41].

## Diabetes

The prevalence of diabetes in the United States is increasing rapidly, as is the incidence of abnormal glucose tolerance, likely driven by the increasing frequency of obesity and sedentary lifestyles. Both individuals with impaired glucose tolerance and those with frank diabetes are at high risk for cardiovascular disorders. Patients with diabetes are at increased risk of cardiovascular disease and also have an increased risk of cardiac events once the diagnosis of CAD has been established. The prevalence of, incidence of, and mortality from all forms of CVD are two- to eightfold higher in persons with diabetes than in those without diabetes [35]. In fact, the projected cardiovascular mortality of a diabetic without known CAD is equivalent to that of a nondiabetic patient who has experienced a myocardial infarction, thus leading to the designation of diabetes as a "coronary risk equivalent." Additional cardiac risk factors amplify the risk in patients with diabetes.

This increased risk impacts both preventive and therapeutic strategies for patients with diabetes and angina. Treatment of other cardiac risk factors, especially hypertension and hyperlipidemia, should be vigorous. Target LDL cholesterol should be less than 100 mg/dL and preferably less than 70 mg/dL [42]. Intensive drug therapy is clearly protective in diabetic patients, and thus all diabetics should therefore have their blood pressure lowered to 135/85 mmHg [25]. Results from the recent ACCORD study were disappointing in that, even more aggressive blood pressure lowering in diabetic patients did not provide incremental benefit, and was associated with more adverse drug reactions [43].

Tight glycemic control is equally important. In patients with type 1 diabetes, the prospective Diabetes Control and Complications Trial showed that strict glycemic control with intensive insulin therapy can both delay the onset of microvascular complications and slow progression of complications already present [44]. Cardiovascular events were decreased from 5.4 to 3.2%, but this did not reach statistical significance [44]. In type II diabetics, the United Kingdom Prospective Diabetes Study also showed a reduced risk of microvascular disease with strict glycemic control [45].

## Exercise

Regular physical activity prevents the development of CAD and reduces symptoms in patients with established cardiovascular disease. The most recent guidelines have extended the recommendations on physical activity to 30–60 min, 7 days per week (minimum 5 days per week). Patients should work toward moderate to intense aerobic activity, with achievement of 80–85% of maximum predicted heart rate and consider resistance training as they become more physically fit. Physical activity reduces insulin resistance, improves glucose intolerance and lipid profiles, and is an important adjunct to diet for achieving and maintaining weight loss.

Comprehensive, exercise-based cardiac rehabilitation reduces mortality rates in patients after myocardial infarction, although the rate of recurrent infarction is not significantly altered. Regular exercise in patients with stable coronary artery disease has been shown to improve myocardial perfusion and to retard disease progression [46]. In fact, it has been demonstrated in a randomized trial of patients with angiographic coronary disease, that compared with percutaneous intervention, a 12-month program of regular physical exercise resulted in superior event-free survival and exercise capacity in selected patients with stable coronary artery disease [47].

## Education

Education is of clear importance to optimize the efficacy of therapeutic and preventive measures. This is as true for physicians and other health workers as it is for the patients themselves. In addition to published literature and patient education materials, a number of web sites, including those of the American College of Cardiology (www.acc.org), the American Heart Association (www.americanheart. org), and the National Institute of Heart, Lung, and Blood (www.nhlbi.nih.gov) provide useful resources.

## Revascularization

If anginal symptoms persist despite maximal medical therapy, coronary angiography with an aim toward possible revascularization should be considered. One must keep in mind that coronary angiography is not a therapeutic intervention, but a diagnostic test. Angiography is of little tangible value if there are no viable revascularization options.

Revascularization can be performed by coronary artery bypass grafting (CABG), in which autologous arteries or veins are used to reroute blood around relatively long segments of the proximal coronary artery, or percutaneous coronary intervention (PCI), a technique that uses catheter-borne mechanical devices to open a (usually) short area of stenosis from within the coronary artery, nowadays usually including implantation of a coronary stent. Both strategies have strengths and weaknesses, and which one would be optimal for a given patient is not always entirely clear. Studies comparing the two may be limited either by a lack of long-term follow-up, or by the "shifting sand" phenomenon, when long-term follow-up has been achieved, but by the time the study is completed, treatments in both arms may have evolved to the point where the trial is not felt to be entirely relevant to contemporary practice.

Revascularization may be chosen to alleviate symptoms or to prolong life expectancy. Among patients with stable angina, the decision to proceed with revascularization is usually made in one of three situations: patients with anatomy for which revascularization has a proven survival benefit, those with activity-limiting symptoms despite maximum medical therapy, and active patients who want PCI for improved quality of life compared to medical therapy.

The benefits of coronary revascularization in reducing cardiac events and death have been widely accepted in the context of acute coronary syndromes with ST-segment elevation MI and non-ST-segment elevation MI [48]. When it comes to chronic stable angina, the benefits of revascularization therapy are much more complicated, and careful patient selection is necessary when considering each therapeutic approach.

The Coronary Artery Surgery Study (CASS) compared surgery to angioplasty by coronary anatomy. On the basis of that trial, there is little doubt that surgery is preferred over medical treatment for patients with significant (>50%) left main stenosis, with an increase in median survival from 6.6 to 13.3 years [49]. Patients with diffuse triple vessel disease and impaired left ventricular function (ejection fraction <50%) also appear to benefit from bypass surgery. Left main equivalent disease, defined as proximal LAD and left circumflex disease (>70%), appears to behave similarly.

Patients with proximal LAD disease and significant disease in one other vessel also appear to derive a mortality benefit from CABG [50].

The 2002 American Heart Association/American College of Cardiology management guidelines recommend coronary revascularization for symptom relief in patients with refractory symptoms despite optimal medical treatment. Revascularization is also indicated for survival benefit in patients deemed to be at high risk of death based on either noninvasive testing (moderate to large areas of reversible ischemia with or without LV dysfunction) or coronary angiography (obstructive left main coronary artery, proximal left anterior descending artery, or three-vessel disease) [35, 39].

In patients without surgical anatomy, the indication for revascularization is relief of symptoms. Factors favoring surgery include high-risk anatomy and unfavorable lesion morphology. Factors favoring PCI include significant comorbidities, particular pulmonary and other factors that may shorten life expectancy. Both percutaneous and surgical techniques are evolving. Drug-eluting stents have reduced restenosis after PCI. Surgical techniques, particularly with respect to the use of arterial conduits and off-pump bypass procedures, are improving as well.

High-risk patients should have a discussion with the cardiothoracic surgeon and interventional cardiologist about the potential operative risks of CABG vs. the technical feasibility of PCI. The benefits and risks involved with each of the options should be clearly laid out before a decision is reached. Multivessel PCI is associated with fewer procedural complications, but also tends to be less durable and associated with a greater number of future procedures. There is little evidence to support a mortality benefit with multivessel PCI in these vulnerable patients. CABG, on the other hand, has a higher procedural risk, especially in patients with multiple comorbidities, but is associated with a more sustained reduction in symptoms, and particularly in the setting of type II diabetes mellitus (and possibly left ventricular dysfunction), has a better overall mortality when an internal mammary artery was utilized as a conduit [51–54]. As technology advances, and as more data become available, the gap between CABG and PCI may narrow.

In patients without specific clinical or angiographic characteristics suggestive of mortality benefit, there is less evidence to support revascularization as opposed to optimal medical management. Two recent meta-analyses showed no mortality benefit with PCI for non-acute coronary artery disease [55, 56]. These data are further supported by the COURAGE trial, which randomly assigned 2,287 nonsurgical patients with objective evidence of ischemia and one or two vessel obstructive CAD to either optimal medical therapy or PCI. Optimal medical therapy was aggressive and included a protocolized approach to antiplatelet and antianginal therapy, lipid management, glucose control, smoking cessation, exercise, and weight reduction. While initially the PCI group fared better with regards to symptom control, after 5 years there was no statistical difference in either the composite endpoint of death and nonfatal MI, or in anginal symptoms [57]. This trial emphasizes the importance – and potential benefits – of aggressive medical therapy for patients with angina. Revascularization should be considered only when patients remain symptomatic despite optima medical therapy, and even then, adjunctive risk factor reduction remains crucial.

# References

1. Lloyd-Jones D, Adams R, Carnethon M, et al. Heart disease and stroke statistics – 2009 update: a report from the American Heart Association Statistics Committee and Stroke Statistics Subcommittee. Circulation. 2009;119:480–6.
2. Braunwald E. Control of myocardial oxygen consumption. Physiologic and clinical considerations. Am J Cardiol. 1971;27:416–32.
3. DeWood MA, Stifter WF, Simpson CS, et al. Coronary arteriographic findings soon after non-Q-wave myocardial infarction. N Engl J Med. 1986;315:417–23.
4. Heberden N. Some account of a disorder of the breast. Med Transactions. 1772;2:59–67.
5. Swap CJ, Nagurney JT. Value and limitations of chest pain history in the evaluation of patients with suspected acute coronary syndromes. JAMA. 2005;294:2623–9.
6. Diamond GA. A clinically relevant classification of chest discomfort. J Am Coll Cardiol. 1983;1:574–5.
7. Voskuil JH, Cramer MJ, Breumelhof R, Timmer R, Smout AJ. Prevalence of esophageal disorders in patients with chest pain newly referred to the cardiologist. Chest. 1996;109: 1210–4.
8. Douglas PS, Khandheria B, Stainback RF, et al. ACCF/ASE/ACEP/AHA/ASNC/SCAI/ SCCT/SCMR 2008 appropriateness criteria for stress echocardiography: a report of the American College of Cardiology Foundation Appropriateness Criteria Task Force, American Society of Echocardiography, American College of Emergency Physicians, American Heart Association, American Society of Nuclear Cardiology, Society for Cardiovascular Angiography and Interventions, Society of Cardiovascular Computed Tomography, and Society for Cardiovascular Magnetic Resonance endorsed by the Heart Rhythm Society and the Society of Critical Care Medicine. J Am Coll Cardiol. 2008;51:1127–47.
9. Hendel RC, Berman DS, Di Carli MF, et al. ACCF/ASNC/ACR/AHA/ASE/SCCT/SCMR/ SNM 2009 Appropriate Use Criteria for Cardiac Radionuclide Imaging: A Report of the American College of Cardiology Foundation Appropriate Use Criteria Task Force, the American Society of Nuclear Cardiology, the American College of Radiology, the American Heart Association, the American Society of Echocardiography, the Society of Cardiovascular Computed Tomography, the Society for Cardiovascular Magnetic Resonance, and the Society of Nuclear Medicine. J Am Coll Cardiol. 2009;53:2201–29.
10. Craven L. Experience with aspirin (acetysalicylic acid) in the non-specific prophylaxis of coronary thrombosis. Miss Vlly Med J. 1953;75:38–44.
11. Lewis Jr HD, Davis JW, Archibald DG, et al. Protective effects of aspirin against acute myocardial infarction and death in men with unstable angina. Results of a Veterans Administration cooperative study. N Engl J Med. 1983;309:396–403.
12. Theroux P, Ouimet H, McCans J, et al. Aspirin, heparin, or both to treat acute unstable angina. N Engl J Med. 1988;319:1105–11.
13. Steering Committee of the Physicians' Health Study Research Group. Final report on the aspirin component of the ongoing physicians' health study. N Engl J Med. 1989;321:129–35.
14. Platelet Receptor Inhibition in Ischemic Syndrome Management in Patients Limited by Unstable Signs and Symptoms (PRISM-PLUS) Study Investigators. Inhibition of the platelet glycoprotein IIb/IIIa receptor with tirofiban in unstable angina and non-Q-wave myocardial infarction. N Engl J Med. 1998;338:1488–97.
15. Ridker PM, Cushman M, Stampfer MJ, Tracy RP, Hennekens CH. Inflammation, aspirin, and the risk of cardiovascular disease in apparently healthy men. N Engl J Med. 1997;336:973–9.
16. CAPRIE Steering Committee. A randomised, blinded, trial of clopidogrel versus aspirin in patients at risk of ischaemic events (CAPRIE). Lancet. 1996;348:1329–39.
17. Cohn PF, Gorlin R. Physiologic and clinical actions of nitroglycerin. Med Clin North Am. 1974;58:407–15.
18. Lacoste LL, Theroux P, Lidon RM, Colucci R, Lam JY. Antithrombotic properties of transdermal nitroglycerin in stable angina pectoris. Am J Cardiol. 1994;73:1058–62.

19. Silber S. Nitrates: why and how should they be used today? Current status of the clinical usefulness of nitroglycerin, isosorbide dinitrate and isosorbide-5-mononitrate. Eur J Clin Pharmacol. 1990;38 Suppl 1:S35–51.
20. Frishman WH. Multifactorial actions of beta-adrenergic blocking drugs in ischemic heart disease: current concepts. Circulation. 1983;67:I11–8.
21. Oliva PB, Potts DE, Pluss RG. Coronary arterial spasm in Prinzmetal angina. Documentation by coronary arteriography. N Engl J Med. 1973;288:745–51.
22. Stason WB, Schmid CH, Niedzwiecki D, et al. Safety of nifedipine in angina pectoris: a meta-analysis. Hypertension. 1999;33:24–31.
23. Wilson SR, Scirica BM, Braunwald E, et al. Efficacy of ranolazine in patients with chronic angina observations from the randomized, double-blind, placebo-controlled MERLIN-TIMI (metabolic efficiency with ranolazine for less ischemia in non-ST-segment elevation acute coronary syndromes) 36 trial. J Am Coll Cardiol. 2009;53:1510–6.
24. Neal B, MacMahon S, Chapman N. Effects of ACE inhibitors, calcium antagonists, and other blood-pressure-lowering drugs: results of prospectively designed overviews of randomised trials. Blood Pressure Lowering Treatment Trialists' Collaboration. Lancet. 2000;356:1955–64.
25. Chobanian AV, Bakris GL, Black HR, et al. Seventh report of the Joint National Committee on Prevention, Detection, Evaluation, and Treatment of High Blood Pressure. Hypertension. 2003;42:1206–52.
26. Lloyd-Jones DM, Hong Y, Labarthe D, et al. Defining and setting national goals for cardiovascular health promotion and disease reduction: the American Heart Association's strategic Impact Goal through 2020 and beyond. Circulation. 2010;121:586–613.
27. Yusuf S, Sleight P, Pogue J, et al. Effects of an angiotensin-converting-enzyme inhibitor, ramipril, on cardiovascular events in high-risk patients. N Engl J Med. 2000;342:145–53.
28. Fox KM. Efficacy of perindopril in reduction of cardiovascular events among patients with stable coronary artery disease: randomised, double-blind, placebo-controlled, multicentre trial (the EUROPA study). Lancet. 2003;362:782–8.
29. Braunwald E, Domanski MJ, Fowler SE, et al. Angiotensin-converting-enzyme inhibition in stable coronary artery disease. N Engl J Med. 2004;351:2058–68.
30. Lipid Research Clinics Program. The lipid research clinics coronary primary prevention trial results. II. The relationship of reduction in incidence of coronary heart disease to cholesterol lowering. JAMA. 1984;251:365–74.
31. Frick MH, Elo O, Haapa K, et al. Helsinki heart study: primary-prevention trial with gemfibrozil in middle-aged men with dyslipidemia. Safety of treatment, changes in risk factors, and incidence of coronary heart disease. N Engl J Med. 1987;317:1237–45.
32. Scandinavian Simvastatin Survival Study Group. Randomised trial of cholesterol lowering in 4444 patients with coronary heart disease: the Scandinavian Simvastatin Survival Study (4S). Lancet. 1994;344:1383–9.
33. Sacks FM, Pfeffer MA, Moye LA, et al. The effect of pravastatin on coronary events after myocardial infarction in patients with average cholesterol levels. N Engl J Med. 1996;335:1001–9.
34. Long-Term Intervention with Pravastatin in Ischaemic Disease (LIPID) Study Group. Prevention of cardiovascular events and death with pravastatin in patients with coronary heart disease and a broad range of initial cholesterol levels. N Engl J Med. 1998;339:1349–57.
35. Gibbons RJ, Abrams J, Chatterjee K, et al. ACC/AHA 2002 guideline update for the management of patients with chronic stable angina–summary article: a report of the American College of Cardiology/American Heart Association Task Force on Practice Guidelines (Committee on the Management of Patients With Chronic Stable Angina). Circulation. 2003;107:149–58.
36. Grundy SM, Cleeman JI, Merz CN, et al. Implications of recent clinical trials for the National Cholesterol Education Program Adult Treatment Panel III guidelines. Circulation. 2004;110:227–39.
37. Cannon CP, Braunwald E, McCabe CH, et al. Intensive versus moderate lipid lowering with statins after acute coronary syndromes. N Engl J Med. 2004;350:1495–504.

38. Nissen SE, Tuzcu EM, Schoenhagen P, et al. Effect of intensive compared with moderate lipid-lowering therapy on progression of coronary atherosclerosis: a randomized controlled trial. JAMA. 2004;291:1071–80.
39. Fraker Jr TD, Fihn SD, Gibbons RJ, et al. 2007 chronic angina focused update of the ACC/AHA 2002 guidelines for the management of patients with chronic stable angina: a report of the American College of Cardiology/American Heart Association Task Force on Practice Guidelines Writing Group to develop the focused update of the 2002 guidelines for the management of patients with chronic stable angina. J Am Coll Cardiol. 2007;50:2264–74.
40. Ockene IS, Miller NH. Cigarette smoking, cardiovascular disease, and stroke: a statement for healthcare professionals from the American Heart Association. American Heart Association Task Force on Risk Reduction. Circulation. 1997;96:3243–7.
41. Krauss RM, Eckel RH, Howard B, et al. AHA Dietary Guidelines: revision 2000: A statement for healthcare professionals from the Nutrition Committee of the American Heart Association. Circulation. 2000;102:2284–99.
42. Lichtenstein AH, Appel LJ, Brands M, et al. Diet and lifestyle recommendations revision 2006: a scientific statement from the American Heart Association Nutrition Committee. Circulation. 2006;114:82–96.
43. Cushman WC, Evans GW, Byington RP, et al. Effects of intensive blood-pressure control in type 2 diabetes mellitus. N Engl J Med. 2010;362:1575–85.
44. Diabetes Control and Complications Trial Research Group. The effect of intensive treatment of diabetes on the development and progression of long-term complications in insulin-dependent diabetes mellitus. N Engl J Med. 1993;329:977–86.
45. UK Prospective Diabetes Study (UKPDS) Group. Intensive blood-glucose control with sulphonylureas or insulin compared with conventional treatment and risk of complications in patients with type 2 diabetes. Lancet. 1998;352:837–53.
46. Thompson PD, Buchner D, Pina IL, et al. Exercise and physical activity in the prevention and treatment of atherosclerotic cardiovascular disease: a statement from the Council on Clinical Cardiology (Subcommittee on Exercise, Rehabilitation, and Prevention) and the Council on Nutrition, Physical Activity, and Metabolism (Subcommittee on Physical Activity). Circulation. 2003;107:3109–16.
47. Hambrecht R, Walther C, Mobius-Winkler S, et al. Percutaneous coronary angioplasty compared with exercise training in patients with stable coronary artery disease: a randomized trial. Circulation. 2004;109:1371–8.
48. Patel MR, Dehmer GJ, Hirshfeld JW, Smith PK, Spertus JA. ACCF/SCAI/STS/AATS/AHA/ASNC 2009 Appropriateness Criteria for Coronary Revascularization: a report by the American College of Cardiology Foundation Appropriateness Criteria Task Force, Society for Cardiovascular Angiography and Interventions, Society of Thoracic Surgeons, American Association for Thoracic Surgery, American Heart Association, and the American Society of Nuclear Cardiology Endorsed by the American Society of Echocardiography, the Heart Failure Society of America, and the Society of Cardiovascular Computed Tomography. J Am Coll Cardiol. 2009;53:530–53.
49. CASS Principal Investigators. Coronary artery surgery study (CASS): a randomized trial of coronary artery bypass surgery. Survival data. Circulation. 1983;68:939–50.
50. European Coronary Surgery Study Group. Prospective randomised study of coronary artery bypass surgery in stable angina pectoris. Lancet. 1980;2:491–5.
51. Frye RL, August P, Brooks MM, et al. A randomized trial of therapies for type 2 diabetes and coronary artery disease. N Engl J Med. 2009;360:2503–15.
52. BARI Investigators. The final 10-year follow-up results from the BARI randomized trial. J Am Coll Cardiol. 2007;49:1600–6.
53. Serruys PW, Morice MC, Kappetein AP, et al. Percutaneous coronary intervention versus coronary-artery bypass grafting for severe coronary artery disease. N Engl J Med. 2009;360:961–72.
54. Comparison of coronary bypass surgery with angioplasty in patients with multivessel disease. The Bypass Angioplasty Revascularization Investigation (BARI) Investigators. N Engl J Med 1996;335:217–25.

55. Katritsis DG, Ioannidis JP. Percutaneous coronary intervention versus conservative therapy in nonacute coronary artery disease: a meta-analysis. Circulation. 2005;111:2906–12.
56. Trikalinos TA, Alsheikh-Ali AA, Tatsioni A, Nallamothu BK, Kent DM. Percutaneous coronary interventions for non-acute coronary artery disease: a quantitative 20-year synopsis and a network meta-analysis. Lancet. 2009;373:911–8.
57. Boden WE, O'Rourke RA, Teo KK, et al. Optimal medical therapy with or without PCI for stable coronary disease. N Engl J Med. 2007;356:1503–16.

# Chapter 2
# Acute Coronary Syndromes

## Definition

Acute coronary syndromes (ACS) describe the spectrum of disease in patients who present with clinical symptoms compatible with acute myocardial ischemia. ACS are a family of disorders that share similar pathogenic mechanisms and represent different points along a common continuum. These syndromes are caused by recent thrombus formation on preexisting coronary artery plaque leading to impaired myocardial oxygen supply. In this sense they differ from stable angina, which is usually precipitated by increased myocardial oxygen demand (e.g. exertion, fever, tachycardia) with background coronary artery narrowing (limitation of oxygen supply).

ACS have traditionally been classified into Q-wave myocardial infarction, non-Q wave myocardial infarction (NQMI), and unstable angina. More recently, classification has shifted and has become based on the initial electrocardiogram (ECG): patients are divided into three groups: those with ST-elevation (ST elevation myocardial infarction, STEMI), without ST elevation but with enzymatic evidence of myocardial damage (non-ST elevation MI, or NSTEMI), and those with unstable angina. Classification according to presenting ECG coincides with current treatment strategies, since patients presenting with ST elevation benefit from immediate reperfusion and should be treated with urgent revascularization or fibrinolytic therapy. Fibrinolytic agents have been shown to be ineffective in other patients with ACS. The discussion in this chapter will follow this schematization.

## Pathophysiology

Myocardial ischemia results from an imbalance between oxygen supply and demand, and usually develops in the setting of obstructive atherosclerotic coronary artery disease, which limits blood supply. The pathophysiology of unstable coronary syndromes and myocardial infarction (MI) usually involves dynamic, partial or complete

S. Hollenberg and S. Heitner, *Cardiology in Family Practice: A Practical Guide*,
Current Clinical Practice 1, DOI 10.1007/978-1-61779-385-1_2,
© Springer Science+Business Media, LLC 2012

occlusion of an epicardial coronary artery because of acute intracoronary thrombus formation.

The common link between the various ACS is the rupture of a vulnerable, but previously quiescent, coronary atherosclerotic plaque [1].

Atherosclerotic plaques are composed of a lipid core, which includes cholesterol, oxidized low-density lipoproteins (LDL), macrophages, and smooth muscle cells, covered by a fibrous cap. Plaque rupture occurs when external mechanical forces exceed the tensile strength of the fibrous cap. After plaque rupture, the clinical consequences depend largely on the balance between prothrombotic and antithrombotic forces [2]. The lipid core contains tissue factor and other thrombogenic materials that lead to platelet activation and aggregation. Fibrinolytic factors such as tissue-plasminogen activator (t-PA), prostacyclin, and nitric oxide act to counteract the potential for thrombosis. Possible sequelae of plaque rupture include thrombus formation with total occlusion, with likely development of STEMI, dissolution of thrombus and healing of the fissure, with clinical stabilization, and subtotal occlusion, which can lead to either non-STEMI or unstable angina. A major factor in the outcome of plaque rupture is blood flow. With subtotal occlusion, high-grade stenosis, or vasospasm, thrombus begins to propagate downstream in the arterial lumen. In contrast to the initial thrombi, which are platelet rich, these thrombi contain large numbers of red cells enmeshed in a web of fibrin. The relative fibrin and platelet content of these lesions vary, with unstable angina/NSTEMI more often associated with platelet-rich lesions and STEMI associated with fibrin-rich clot, although it should be noted that all lesions contain some degree of both components [2]. The former would be expected to respond best to antiplatelet therapy, the latter to antithrombotic and fibrinolytic therapy.

## Diagnosis

### Signs and Symptoms

Patients with myocardial ischemia can present with chest pain or pressure, shortness of breath, palpitations, syncope, or sudden death. The pain of myocardial infarction is typically severe, constant, and retrosternal. The pain commonly spreads across the chest and may radiate to the throat or jaw, or down the arms. Its duration is most often more than 20 min. Diaphoresis, nausea, pallor, and anxiety are often present. Prodromal symptoms of myocardial ischemia occur in 20–60% of patients in the days preceding the infarct. The pain of unstable angina may be similar, although it is often milder.

Although these are the classic signs of infarction, it is important to recognize that the pain of myocardial infarction may sometimes be atypical in terms of location or perception. It may be epigastric, confined to the jaw, arms, wrists, or interscapular region, or perceived as burning or pressure.

The physical examination can be insensitive and nonspecific, but is useful in diagnosing specific complications and in excluding alternative diagnoses, both cardiovascular (such as aortic dissection or pericarditis) and non-cardiac. Distended jugular veins signal right ventricular diastolic pressure elevation, and the appearance of pulmonary crackles (in the absence of pulmonary disease) indicates elevated left ventricular filling pressures. Left ventricular failure is suggested by the presence of basal crackles, tachycardia, and tachypnea, and an S3 gallop, which usually indicates a large infarction with extensive muscle damage. A systolic murmur of mitral regurgitation may be present due to papillary muscle dysfunction or LV dilation. A pansystolic murmur may also result from an acute ventricular septal defect due to septal rupture.

## The Electrocardiogram

The ECG abnormalities in myocardial ischemia depend on the extent and nature of coronary stenosis and the presence of collateral flow, but the pattern of ECG changes generally gives a guide to the area and extent of infarction (see Table 2.1). The number of leads involved broadly reflects the extent of myocardium involved.

Table 2.1 Localization of myocardial infarction by electrocardiography

| Area of infarction | ECG leads | Infarct-related artery |
|---|---|---|
| Inferior | II, III, aVF | RCA or posterolateral branch of Cx |
| Anterior | V2–V4 | LAD or diagonal branch of LAD |
| Lateral | I, aVL, V5, V6 | Cx |
| True posterior | Tall R wave in V1 | Posterolateral branch of Cx or posterior descending branch of RCA |
| Septal | V1–V3 | LAD or diagonal branch of LAD |
| Anterolateral | I, aVL, V2–V6 | Proximal LAD |
| Inferolateral | II, III, aVF, I, aVL, V5, V6 | Proximal Cx or large RCA in right dominant system |
| Right ventricular | V3R, V4R | RCA |

*RCA* right coronary artery; *LAD* left anterior descending coronary artery; *Cx* circumflex coronary artery

With acute total acute occlusion of a coronary artery, the first demonstrable ECG changes are peaked T waves changes in the leads reflecting the anatomic area of myocardium in jeopardy. As total occlusion continues, there is elevation of the ST segments in the same leads. With continued occlusion, there is an evolution of ECG abnormalities, with biphasic and then inverted T waves. If enough myocardium is infarcted, Q waves may appear. These represent unopposed initial depolarization forces away from the mass of infarcted myocardium, which has lost electrical activity and no longer contributes to the mean QRS voltage vector. The formation of Q waves is accompanied by a decrease in the magnitude of the R waves in the same leads, representing diminution of voltage in the mass of infarcted myocardium.

Indeed, loss of R wave voltage, revealed by comparison with previous ECG tracings, may be the only ECG evidence for the presence of permanent myocardial damage.

Extension of an inferior MI to the posterior segment can be detected by enhancement of R waves in the anterior chest leads, since these forces are now less balanced by opposite posterior forces. True posterior infarction can be subtle, since the only signs may be prominent R waves, tall upright T waves and depressed ST segments in leads $V_1$ and $V_2$. Involvement of the right ventricle in inferior MI is also not readily detected on the standard 12-lead ECG because of the small mass of the right ventricle relative to the left ventricle and because of the positioning of the standard precordial leads away from the right ventricle. RV infarction may be detected by ST elevation in recordings from right precordial leads, particularly $V_{4R}$ [3].

A number of potential pitfalls can contribute to misinterpretation of the ECG. Many conditions can mimic STEMI and lead to false positives. Early repolarization pattern with up to 3 mm ST elevation in leads V1–V3 can be seen in healthy individuals, usually young men. Pre-excitation, bundle branch block, pericarditis, pulmonary embolism, subarachnoid hemorrhage, metabolic disturbances such as hyperkalemia, hypothermia, and LV aneurysm can be associated with ST elevation in the absence of acute myocardial ischemia. In pericarditis, ST segments may be elevated, but the elevation is diffuse and the morphology of the ST segments in pericarditis tends to be concave upward, while that of ischemia is convex. Pericarditis may also be distinguished from infarction by the presence of PR segment depression in the inferior leads (and also by PR segment in lead aVR) [4]. On the other hand, some conditions can lead to false negatives, including prior myocardial infarction, paced rhythm, and left bundle branch block (LBBB) when acute ischemia is not recognized. These pitfalls are common in the real world and in large clinical trials; when ECG from the GUSTO-IIB trial were reviewed by expert readers at a core lab, 15% of patients with STEMI were found to have been misclassified as NSTEMI, and these patients had a 21% higher mortality [5].

**Cardiac Biomarkers**

Measurement of enzymes released into the serum from necrotic myocardial cells after infarction can aid in the diagnosis of myocardial infarction [6]. The classic biochemical marker of acute myocardial infarction is elevation of the CPK MB isoenzyme. CPK MB begins to appear in the plasma 4–8 h after onset of infarction, peaks at 12–24 h and returns to baseline at 2–4 days. To be diagnostic for MI, the total plasma CPK value must exceed the upper limit of normal, and the MB fraction must exceed a certain value (usually >5%, but depends on the assay used).

These biomarkers have now been superseded by troponin T and I, parts of the troponin-tropomyosin complex in cardiac myocytes [7, 8]. Troponin elevations are highly specific for myocardial cellular injury. Troponin is also much more sensitive than CK-MB as a result of its higher concentration in cardiac muscle, and can detect even minor cardiac injury [8]. Even minor increases in circulating troponin values correlate with adverse outcomes in the short and long term [7]. In non-ST elevation

ACS elevated troponins not only predict increased risk, but also identify the patients most likely to benefit from more aggressive therapeutic strategies [9]. Troponins may not be elevated until 4–6 h after an acute event, and so critical therapeutic interventions should not be delayed pending assay results. Once elevated, troponin levels can remain high for days to weeks, limiting their utility to detect late reinfarction.

## ST Elevation Myocardial Infarction

Symptoms suggestive of MI are usually similar to those of ordinary angina but are greater in intensity and duration. Nausea, vomiting, and diaphoresis may be prominent features, and stupor and malaise attributable to low cardiac output may occur. Compromised left ventricular function may result in pulmonary edema with development of pulmonary bibasilar crackles and jugular venous distention; a fourth heart sound can be present with small infarcts or even mild ischemia, but a third heart sound is usually indicative of more extensive damage.

Patients presenting with suspected myocardial ischemia should undergo a rapid evaluation, and should be treated with oxygen, sublingual nitroglycerin (unless systolic pressure is less than 90 mmHg), adequate analgesia, and aspirin, 160–325 mg orally [9, 10]. Opiates relieve pain, and also reduce anxiety, the salutary effects of which have been known for decades and should not be underestimated. A 12-lead ECG should be performed and interpreted expeditiously.

ST-segment elevation of at least 1 mV in 2 or more contiguous leads provides strong evidence of thrombotic coronary occlusion, the patient should be considered for immediate reperfusion therapy. The diagnosis of STEMI can be limited in the presence of preexisting LBBB or permanent pacemaker. Nonetheless, new LBBB with a compatible clinical presentation should be treated as acute myocardial infarction and treated accordingly. Indeed, recent data suggest that patients with STEMI and new LBBB may stand to gain greater benefit from reperfusion strategies than those with ST elevation and preserved ventricular conduction.

One possible treatment algorithm for treating patients with ST-elevation, MI is shown in Fig. 2.1.

### Thrombolytic Therapy

Early reperfusion of an occluded coronary artery is indicated for all eligible candidates. Overwhelming evidence from multiple clinical trials demonstrates the ability of thrombolytic agents administered early in the course of an acute MI to reduce infarct size, preserve left ventricular function, and reduce short-term and long-term mortality [11, 12]. Patients treated early derive the most benefit, but it is reasonable to administer fibrinolytics to patients who have continued clinical or ECG evidence of ischemia. Indications and contraindications for thrombolytic therapy are listed in Table 2.2.

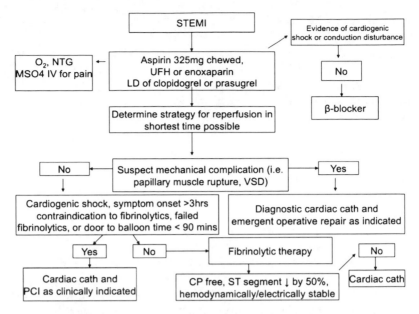

**Fig. 2.1** Treatment algorithm for ST-elevation myocardial infarction. *CP* chest pain; *LD* loading dose; *MSO₄* morphine; *NTG* nitroglycerin; *O₂* oxygen; *UFH* unfractionated heparin; *VSD* ventricular septal defect

**Table 2.2** Indications for and contraindications to thrombolytic therapy in acute myocardial infarction

| |
|---|
| Indications |
|     Symptoms consistent with acute myocardial infarction |
|     ECG showing 1-mm (0.1 mV) ST elevation in at least two contiguous leads, or new left bundle-branch block |
|     Presentation within 12 h of symptom onset |
|     Absence of contraindications |
| Contraindications |
| Absolute |
|     Active internal bleeding |
|     Intracranial neoplasm, aneurysm, or A–V malformation |
|     Stroke or neurosurgery within 6 weeks |
|     Trauma or major surgery within 2 weeks which could be a potential source of serious rebleeding |
|     Aortic dissection |
| Relative |
|     Prolonged (>10 min) or clearly traumatic cardiopulmonary resuscitation[a] |
|     Noncompressible vascular punctures |
|     Severe uncontrolled hypertension (>200/110 mmHg)[a] |
|     Trauma or major surgery within 6 weeks (but more than 2 weeks) |
|     Pre-existing coagulopathy or current use of anticoagulants with INR >2–3 |
|     Active peptic ulcer |
|     Infective endocarditis |
|     Pregnancy |
|     Chronic severe hypertension |

[a]Could be an absolute contraindication in low-risk patients with myocardial infarction

Because of the small, but nonetheless significant, risk of a bleeding complication, most notably intracranial hemorrhage, selection of patients with acute MI for administration of a thrombolytic agent should be undertaken with prudence and caution. High-risk patients are usually better treated with emergent coronary angiography with percutaneous coronary intervention (PCI).

**Thrombolytic Agents**

Streptokinase was the original fibrinolytic agent used in STEMI, but has not been superseded by t-PA, a recombinant protein that is more fibrin-selective than streptokinase and produces a higher early coronary patency rate (70–80%) [13, 14]. t-PA is given in an accelerated regimen consisting of a 15 mg bolus, 0.75 mg/kg (up to 50 mg) IV over the initial 30 min, and 0.5 mg/kg (up to 35 mg) over the next 60 min.

Reteplase (r-PA) is a deletion mutant of t-PA with an extended half-life, and is given as two 10 mg boluses 30 min apart. Reteplase was originally evaluated in angiographic trials that demonstrated improved coronary flow at 90 min compared to t-PA, but subsequent trials showed similar 30-day mortality rates [15].

Tenecteplase (TNK-tPA) is a genetically engineered t-PA mutant with amino acid substitutions that result in prolonged half-life, resistance to plasminogen-activator inhibitor-1, and increased fibrin specificity. TNK-tPA is given as a single bolus, adjusted for weight. A single bolus of TNK-tPA has been shown to produce coronary flow rates identical to those seen with accelerated t-PA, with equivalent 30-day mortality and bleeding rates [16].

Because these newer agents in general have equivalent efficacy and side effect profiles, at no current additional cost compared to t-PA, and because they are simpler to administer, they have gained popularity. An ideal fibrinolytic agent would have greater fibrin specificity, slower clearance from the circulation, and more resistance to plasma protease inhibitors, but has not yet been developed.

## Primary Percutaneous Coronary Intervention in Acute Myocardial Infarction

The major advantages of primary PCI over thrombolytic therapy include a higher rate of normal (TIMI grade 3) flow, lower risk of intracranial hemorrhage and the ability to stratify risk based on the severity and distribution of coronary artery disease. Patients ineligible for fibrinolytic therapy should obviously be considered for primary PCI. In addition, data from several randomized trials have suggested that PCI is preferable to thrombolytic therapy for AMI patients at higher risk [17]. The largest of these trials is the GUSTO-IIB Angioplasty Substudy, which randomized 1,138 patients. At 30 days, there was a clinical benefit in the combined primary endpoints of death, nonfatal reinfarction, and nonfatal disabling stroke in the patients treated with PTCA compared to t-PA, but no difference in the "hard" endpoints of death and myocardial infarction at 30 days [18].

Recent meta-analyses comparing direct PTCA with fibrinolytic therapy have suggested lower rates of mortality and reinfarction among those receiving direct PTCA [19, 20]. Thus, direct angioplasty, if performed in a timely manner (ideally within 60 min) by highly experienced personnel, may be the preferred method of revascularization since it offers more complete revascularization with improved restoration of normal coronary blood flow and detailed information about coronary anatomy [10]. There are certain subpopulations in which primary PCI is clearly preferred, and other populations in which the data are suggestive of benefit. These subsets are listed in Table 2.3.

**Table 2.3** Situations in which primary angioplasty is preferred in acute myocardial infarction

| |
| --- |
| Situations in which PTCA is clearly preferable to thrombolytics |
|   Contraindications to thrombolytic therapy |
|   Cardiogenic shock |
|   Patients in whom uncertain diagnosis prompted cardiac catheterization which revealed coronary occlusion |
| Situations in which PTCA *may be* preferable to thrombolytics |
|   Elderly patients (>75 years) |
|   Hemodynamic instability |
|   Patients with prior coronary artery bypass grafting |
|   Large anterior infarction |
|   Patients with a prior myocardial infarction |

More important than the method of revascularization is the time to revascularization, and that this should be achieved in the most efficient and expeditious manner possible [21]. It is important to keep in mind that early, complete, and sustained reperfusion after myocardial infarction is known to decrease 30-day mortality. The preferred method for reperfusion in STEMI is PCI only, if it can be done within a timely manner. Practical considerations regarding transport to a PCI capable facility should be carefully reviewed before forgoing thrombolytics for PCI. Early recognition and diagnosis of STEMI are key to achieving the desired door-to-needle (or medical contact-to-needle) time for initiation of fibrinolytic therapy of 30 min or door-to-balloon (or medical contact-to-balloon) time for PCI under 90 min [10]. Achieving reperfusion in timely manner correlates with improvement in ultimate infarct size, left ventricular function, and survival [22, 23]. The ultimate goal is to restore adequate blood flow through the infarct-related artery to the infarct zone as well as to limit microvascular damage and reperfusion injury. The latter is accomplished with adjunctive and ancillary treatments that will be discussed below.

## Coronary Stenting

Primary angioplasty for acute myocardial infarction results in a significant reduction in mortality but is limited by the possibility of abrupt vessel closure, recurrent in-hospital ischemia, reocclusion of the infarct-related artery, and restenosis. The use of coronary stents has been shown to reduce restenosis and adverse cardiac outcomes in both routine and high-risk PCI [24]. The PAMI stent trial was designed to test the hypothesis that routine implantation of an intracoronary stent in the setting of myocardial infarction would reduce angiographic restenosis and improve clinical outcomes compared to primary balloon angioplasty alone. This large, randomized, multicenter trial involving 900 patients did not show a difference in mortality at 6 months but did show improvement in ischemia-driven target-vessel revascularization and less angina in the stented patients compared to balloon angioplasty alone [25]. Despite the lack of definite data demonstrating mortality benefit, virtually all of the trials investigating adjunctive therapy for STEMI have employed a strategy of primary stenting, and stenting has become the default strategy. Whether to use a bare metal stent (BMS) or a drug-eluting stent (DES) in acute MI is a question that has not yet been addressed definitively by clinical trials; selection is currently based on both patient and angiographic characteristics.

## Adjunctive Therapies in STEMI

### Aspirin

Aspirin is the best known and the most widely used of all the antiplatelet agents because of low cost and relatively low toxicity. Aspirin inhibits the production of thromboxane A2 by irreversibly acetylating the serine residue of the enzyme prostaglandin $H_2$ synthetase. Aspirin has been shown to reduce mortality in acute infarction to the same degree as fibrinolytic therapy, and its effects are additive to fibrinolytics [26]. In addition, aspirin reduces the risk of reinfarction [27, 28]. Unless contraindicated, all patients with a suspected ACS (STEMI, NSTEMI, unstable angina) should be given aspirin as soon as possible.

### Thienopyridines

Thienopyridines are a class of oral antiplatelet agents that block the P2Y12 component of the adenosine diphosphate receptor and thus inhibit the activation and aggregation of platelets. Currently used thienopyridines include clopidogrel and prasugrel. Clopidogrel is converted in the liver to an active metabolite, and onset of inhibition of platelet aggregation (IPA) is dose-dependent, with a 300–600 mg loading dose achieving inhibition of platelet within 2 h.

Clopidogrel in combination with aspirin was shown to reduce the composite endpoint of infarct artery patency, death, or recurrent MI before angiography when given in conjunction with fibrinolytic therapy, heparin, and aspirin in the 3,491 patient CLARITY TIMI-28 trial [29]. When the 1,863 patients in CLARITY TIMI-28 that underwent PCI were examined, retreatment with clopidogrel in addition to aspirin resulted in a significant reduction in cardiovascular death, MI, or stroke at 30 days (7.5 vs. 12.0%; $p = 0.001$) without causing excess bleeding [30]. It is therefore routine practice to administer a loading dose of clopidogrel 300 or 600 mg prior to PCI.

Prasugrel is a recently approved thienopyridine that irreversibly binds to the P2Y12 component of the ADP receptor with a more rapid onset of action and more complete metabolism to the active metabolite, resulting in a higher level of IPA than clopidogrel. Prasugrel (given as a loading dose of 60 mg followed by maintenance dose of 10 mg in patients without renal insufficiency) decreased the combined endpoint of death, MI, and stroke compared to clopidogrel (300 mg load, followed by 75 mg maintenance) in the randomized, double-blind TRITON-TIMI 38 trial of 13,608 ACS patients undergoing PCI for ACS (3,534 STEMI, 10,074 UA/NSTEMI) [31]. The rate of major bleeding was higher in the prasugrel group, as was the rate of life-threatening bleeding. A post-hoc analysis of the trial showed harm with prasugrel patients with a history of TIA or stroke, and no benefit in patients older than 75 or weighing less than 60 kg, so caution is warranted in these groups [31].

Dual antiplatelet therapy with aspirin and thienopyridines is given to all patients undergoing PCI, as described above. However, data suggest that even patients not undergoing PCI benefit from the addition of clopidogrel to aspirin. In the COMMIT-CCS-2 trial, a broad population of 45,852 unselected patients with ST-elevation MI, only 54% of patients were treated with fibrinolytics, and most of the rest had no revascularization at all [32]. Clopidogrel added to aspirin decreased all-cause mortality from 8.1 to 7.5% ($p = 0.03$), without increased bleeding in the clopidogrel group [32]. On the basis of these data, patients presenting with MI should be considered for a thienopyridine regardless of whether or not they underwent reperfusion therapy. The optimal duration of thienopyridine use in this population has yet to be defined.

**Glycoprotein IIb/IIIa Receptor Antagonists**

Glycoprotein IIb/IIIa receptor antagonists inhibit the final common pathway of platelet aggregation, blocking crosslinking of activated platelets, and are often used in percutaneous intervention [33]. Three agents are currently available. Abciximab is a chimeric murine-human monoclonal antibody Fab fragment with a short plasma half-life (10–30 min) but a long duration of biologic action. Tirofibanis is a small molecule, synthetic nonpeptide agent with a half-life of approximately 2.5 h and a lower receptor affinity than abciximab. Eptifibatide is a small molecule, cyclic heptapeptide with a 2-h half-life.

In the era of dual antiplatelet therapy using a thienopyridine and aspirin, the role of addition of a glycoprotein IIb/IIIa inhibitor in primary angioplasty for STEMI is uncertain. Studies such as the ADMIRAL and CADILLAC trials conducted prior to the use of dual antiplatelet therapy established the efficacy of abciximab in primary PCI (with or without stenting) in patients with STEMI [34, 35]. The results of recent clinical trials have raised questions about whether glycoprotein IIb/IIIa antagonists have additional utility when added to dual antiplatelet therapy in patients with STEMI [36–38]. When either abciximab or placebo was added to 600 mg of clopidogrel randomized 800 patients undergoing primary stenting in the BRAVE-3 trial, there was no difference in either infarct size or the secondary composite endpoint of death, recurrent myocardial infarction, stroke, or urgent revascularization of the infarct-related artery [36]. Similar findings were seen in ON-TIME 2, in which tirofiban added to dual antiplatelet therapy in 984 patients with STEMI prior to transport for PCI improved resolution of ST segment elevation, but did not change the 30 day composite endpoint of death, recurrent MI, or urgent target-vessel revascularization [38]. The current guidelines suggest that when an STEMI patient is treated with a thienopyridine and aspirin plus an anticoagulant such as unfractionated heparin (UFH) or bivalirudin, the use of a glycoprotein IIb/IIIa inhibitor at the time of PCI may be beneficial, but cannot be recommended as routine [10].

## Anticoagulants

Administration of full-dose heparin after thrombolytic therapy with t-PA is essential to diminish reocclusion after successful reperfusion [11, 26]. Dosing should be adjusted to weight, with a bolus of 60 U/kg up to a maximum of 4,000 U and an initial infusion rate of 12 U/kg/h up to a maximum of 1,000 U/h, with adjustment to keep the partial thromboplastin time (PTT) between 50 and 70 s. Heparin should be continued for 24–48 h. For patients undergoing PCI who have already been treated with aspirin and a thienopyridine, both UFH or bivalirudin (with or without prior heparin administration) are acceptable anticoagulant regimens [10].

Enoxaparin is a low-molecular weight heparin (LMWH) with established efficacy as an anticoagulant in patients with STEMI who have received fibrinolytics or are undergoing PCI [39, 40]. The standard dose of enoxaparin is a 30 mg intravenous bolus, followed 15 min later by subcutaneous injections of 1.0 mg/kg every 12 h. Patients with decreased creatinine clearance or those older than 75 are at higher risk of bleeding with standard dose enoxaparin. They should not receive a bolus but can receive a reduced dose of 0.75 mg/kg every 12 h. Patients undergoing PCI should have an additional bolus if the last dose was given 8–12 h prior. Maintenance dosing of enoxaparin should be given during the hospitalization (up to 8 days).

Bivalirudin is 20-amino acid peptide based on the structure of hirudin, a natural anticoagulant isolated from the saliva of the medicinal leech, *Hirudo medicinalis*; bivalirudin is a direct thrombin inhibitor that inhibits both clot-bound and circulating thrombin. It is administered as an initial bolus of 0.75 mg/kg, followed by a continuous infusion at 1.75 mg/kg/h for the duration of PCI, with adjustments for patients with renal dysfunction. Bivalirudin is probably as good as heparin plus a glycoprotein IIb/IIIa inhibitor in reducing ischemic events associated with unstable angina and/or non-ST elevation myocardial infarction (NSTEMI) with the added benefit of a reduction in bleeding [41]. The potential role of bivalirudin in

STEMI was clarified by HORIZONS-AMI trial, which randomized 3,602 patients with STEMI undergoing primary PCI to UFH plus a glycoprotein IIb/IIIa inhibitor or to bivalirudin alone (with provisional glycoprotein IIb/IIIa in the cardiac catheterization lab) [42]. Major adverse cardiac event (MACE) rates were equivalent, but use of bivalirudin alone was associated with a 40% reduction in bleeding [42]. Bivalirudin is also an excellent alternative to unfractionated or LMWH in patients with a history of heparin-induced thrombocytopenia.

## Nitrates

Nitrates have a number of beneficial effects in acute myocardial infarction. They reduce myocardial oxygen demand by decreasing preload and afterload, and may also improve myocardial oxygen supply by increasing subendocardial perfusion and collateral blood flow to the ischemic region [43]. Occasional patients with ST elevation due to occlusive coronary artery spasm may have dramatic resolution of ischemia with nitrates. In addition to their hemodynamic effects, nitrates also reduce platelet aggregation. Despite these benefits, the GISSI-3 and ISIS-4 trials failed to show a significant reduction in mortality from routine acute and chronic nitrate therapies [44, 45]. Nonetheless, nitrates are still first-line agents for the symptomatic relief of angina pectoris and when myocardial infarction is complicated by congestive heart failure.

## Beta Blockers

Beta blockers are beneficial both in the early management of myocardial infarction and as long-term therapy. In the pre-thrombolytic era, early intravenous atenolol was shown to significantly reduce reinfarction, cardiac arrest, cardiac rupture, and death [46]. In conjunction with thrombolytic therapy with t-PA, immediate β-blockade with metoprolol resulted in a significant reduction in recurrent ischemia and reinfarction, although mortality was not decreased [47].

The COMMIT-CCS 2 trial of 45,852 patients with acute MI had a factorial arm (the clopidogrel arm was discussed above) and randomized patients, 93% of whom had STEMI and 54% of whom were treated with lytics, to treatment with metoprolol (three intravenous injections of 5 mg each followed by oral 200 mg/day for up to 4 weeks) or placebo [48]. Surprisingly, there was no difference in the primary endpoint of death, reinfarction, or cardiac arrest by treatment group or in the co-primary endpoint of all-cause mortality by hospital discharge. Although reinfarction was lower in the metoprolol group, there was an increase in the risk of developing heart failure and cardiogenic shock, and death due to shock occurred more frequently in the metoprolol group [48]. Based on these findings, routine use of intravenous beta blockers in the absence of systemic hypertension is no longer recommended [10].

In contrast to the use of early, aggressive beta blocker therapy, the long-term use of beta blockers post-MI has favorable outcomes on mortality [46, 49]. The CArvedilol Post-infaRct survIval COntRolled evaluatioN (CAPRICORN) trial randomized patients with systolic dysfunction already treated with angiotensin-converting enzyme (ACE) inhibitors after MI to carvedilol or placebo, and showed decreased cardiovascular mortality as well as a decrease in the composite outcome of all-cause mortality or nonfatal MI [50]. This study supports the claim that beta blocker therapy after acute MI reduces mortality irrespective of reperfusion therapy or ace inhibitor use. Relative contraindications to oral beta blockers include heart rate less than 60 bpm, systolic arterial pressure less than 100 mmHg, moderate or severe LV failure, signs of peripheral hypoperfusion, shock, PR interval greater than 0.24 s, second or third-degree AV block, active asthma, or reactive airway disease [10]. Diabetes mellitus is not a contraindication.

### Lipid-Lowering Agents

Extensive epidemiologic, laboratory, and clinical evidence provide a convincing relationship linking cholesterol and coronary artery disease. Total cholesterol level has been linked to the development of CAD events with a continuous and graded relation, with a close association with LDL cholesterol [51]. Most of this risk is due to LDL cholesterol. Numerous large primary and secondary prevention trials have shown that LDL cholesterol lowering is associated with a reduced risk of coronary disease events. Earlier lipid-lowering trials used bile-acid sequestrants (cholestyramine), fibric acid derivatives (gemfibrozil and clofibrate), or niacin, in addition to diet, achieving a reduction in total cholesterol of 6–15%, accompanied by a consistent trend toward a reduction in fatal and nonfatal coronary events [52].

HMG-CoA reductase inhibitors (statins) produce larger reductions in cholesterol, with more impressive clinical results. Statins have been demonstrated to decrease the rate of adverse ischemic events and mortality when used both as primary prevention in high-risk patients [53, 54], and as secondary prevention in patients with documented CAD [55–57]. The goal of treatment is an LDL cholesterol level less than 70–100 mg/dL [58], although there appears to be a linear relationship between LDL levels and events, and many clinicians recommend an LDL goal of <70 mg/dL, especially for secondary prevention [59]. Maximum benefit may require management of other lipid abnormalities (elevated triglycerides, low HDL cholesterol) and treatment of other atherogenic risk factors.

### Angiotensin-Converting Enzyme Inhibitors

ACE inhibitors are clearly beneficial in patients with congestive heart failure. ACE inhibitors were shown to decrease mortality in the SAVE trial, in which patients with left ventricular dysfunction (ejection fraction <40%) after MI had a 21% improvement in survival after treatment with the ACE inhibitor captopril [60]. A smaller but still significant reduction in mortality was seen when all patients were treated with captopril in the ISIS-4 study [45]. The mechanisms responsible for the benefits of ACE inhibitors probably include limitation in the progressive left ventricular dysfunction and enlargement (remodeling) that often occur after infarction, but a reduction in ischemic events was seen as well.

ACE inhibition should be started early, preferably within the first 24 h after infarction. Immediate intravenous ACE inhibition with enalaprilat has not been shown to be beneficial [61]. Patients should be started on low doses of oral agents (captopril 6.25 mg thrice daily) and rapidly increased to the range demonstrated beneficial in clinical trials (captopril 50 mg thrice daily, enalapril 10–20 mg twice daily, lisinopril 10–20 mg once daily, or ramipril 10 mg once daily).

## Calcium Channel Blockers

Randomized clinical trials have not demonstrated that routine use of calcium channel blockers improves survival after myocardial infarction. In fact, meta-analyses suggest that high doses of the short-acting dihydropyridine nifedipine increase mortality in myocardial infarction [62]. Adverse effects of calcium channel blockers include bradycardia, atrioventricular block, and exacerbation of heart failure. The relative vasodilating, negative inotropic effects, and conduction system effects of the various agents must be considered when they are employed in this setting. Diltiazem is the only calcium channel blocker that has been proven to have tangible benefits, reducing reinfarction and recurrent ischemia in patients with non-Q-wave infarctions who do not have evidence of congestive heart failure [63].

Calcium channel blockers may be useful for patients whose postinfarction course is complicated by recurrent angina, because these agents not only reduce myocardial oxygen demand but also inhibit coronary vasoconstriction. For hemodynamically stable patients, diltiazem can be given, starting at 60–90 mg orally every 6–8 h. In patients with severe left ventricular dysfunction, long-acting dihydropyridines without prominent negative inotropic effects such as amlodipine, nicardipine, or the long-acting preparation of nifedipine may be preferable; increased mortality with these agents has not been demonstrated.

## Antiarrhythmic Therapy

A major purpose for admitting MI patients to the ICU is to monitor for and prevent malignant arrhythmias. Ventricular extrasystoles are common after MI and are a manifestation of electrical instability of peri-infarct areas. The incidence of sustained ventricular tachycardia or fibrillation is highest in the first 3–4 h, but these arrhythmias may occur at any time. Malignant ventricular arrhythmias may be heralded by frequent premature ventricular contractions (PVCs), complex ectopy (couplets, multiform PVCs), and salvos of nonsustained ventricular tachycardia. However, malignant arrhythmia may occur suddenly without these preceding "warning" arrhythmias. Based on these pathophysiologic considerations, prophylactic use of intravenous lidocaine even in the absence of ectopy has been advocated, but even though lidocaine decreases the frequency of PVCs and of early ventricular fibrillation, overall mortality is not decreased. In fact, meta-analyses of pooled data have demonstrated increased mortality from the routine use of lidocaine [64], and so its routine prophylactic administration is no longer recommended [10].

Lidocaine infusion may be used after an episode of sustained ventricular tachycardia or ventricular fibrillation, and might be considered in patients with nonsustained ventricular tachycardia. Lidocaine is administered as a bolus of 1 mg/kg (not to exceed 100 mg), followed by a second bolus of 0.5 mg/kg, 10 min later, along with an infusion at 1–3 mg/min. Lidocaine is metabolized by the liver, and so lower doses should be given in the presence of liver disease, in the elderly, and in patients who have congestive heart failure severe enough to compromise hepatic perfusion. Toxic manifestations primarily involve the central nervous system, and can include confusion, lethargy, slurred speech, and seizures. Because the risk of malignant ventricular arrhythmias decreases after 24 h, lidocaine is usually discontinued after this point. For prolonged infusions, monitoring of lidocaine levels (therapeutic between 1.5 and 5 g/mL) is occasionally useful.

Intravenous amiodarone is an alternative to lidocaine for ventricular arrhythmias. Amiodarone is given as a 150 mg IV bolus over 10 min, followed by 1 mg/min for 6 h, then 0.5 mg/min for 18 h.

Perhaps the most important point in the prevention and management of arrhythmias after acute myocardial infarction is correcting hypoxemia, and maintaining normal serum potassium and magnesium levels. Serum electrolytes should be followed closely, particularly after diuretic therapy. Magnesium depletion is also a frequently overlooked cause of persistent ectopy [65]. The serum magnesium level, even if it is within normal limits, may not reflect myocardial concentrations. Routine administration of magnesium has not been shown to reduce mortality after acute myocardial infarction [45], but empiric administration of 2 g of intravenous magnesium in patients with early ventricular ectopy is probably a good idea.

## Non-ST Elevation Myocardial Infarction

The key to initial management of patients with ACS without ST elevation is risk stratification. The overall risk of a patient is related to both the severity of preexisting heart disease and the degree of plaque instability. Risk stratification is an ongoing process, which begins with hospital admission and continues through discharge.

Braunwald has proposed a classification for unstable angina based on severity of symptoms and clinical circumstances for risk stratification [66]. The risk of progression to acute MI or death in ACS increases with age. ST segment depression on the ECG identifies patients at higher risk for clinical events [66]. Conversely, a normal ECG confers an excellent short-term prognosis. Biochemical markers of cardiac injury are also predictive of outcome. Elevated levels of troponin T are associated with an increased risk of cardiac events and a higher 30-day mortality, and in fact, were more strongly correlated with 30-day survival than ECG category or CPK

MB level in an analysis of data from the GUSTO-II trial [67]. Conversely, low levels are associated with low event rates, although the absence of troponin elevation does not guarantee a good prognosis and is not a substitute for good clinical judgment.

## Antiplatelet Therapy

As previously noted, aspirin is a mainstay of therapy for ACS. Both the VA Cooperative Study Group [27] and the Canadian multicenter trial [68] showed that aspirin reduces the risk of death or myocardial infarction by approximately 50% in patients with unstable angina or NQMI. Aspirin also reduces events after resolution of an ACS, and should be continued indefinitely.

As in patients with STEMI, patients with NSTEMI have been shown to benefit from the use of a thienopyridine in addition to aspirin. In the CURE trial, 12,562 patients were randomized to receive clopidogrel or placebo in addition to standard therapy with aspirin, within 24 h of unstable angina symptoms [69]. Clopidogrel significantly reduced the risk of myocardial infarction, stroke, or cardiovascular death from 11.4 to 9.3% ($p < 0.001$) [69]. It should be noted that this benefit came with a 1% absolute increase in major, non-life threatening bleeds ($p = 0.001$) as well as a 2.8% absolute increase in major/life-threatening bleeds associated with CABG within 5 days ($p = 0.07$) [69]. Because percutaneous revascularization was performed on only 23% of patients in the CURE trial during the initial hospitalization, the study provides convincing evidence that clopidogrel is beneficial in patients who are managed medically in addition to those undergoing PCI.

The TRITON-TIMI 38 trial comparing prasugrel to clopidogrel included 10,074 UA/NSTEMI patients as well as 3,534 STEMI patients [31]. The primary endpoint – cardiovascular death, nonfatal MI, and nonfatal stroke – was significantly lower in the prasugrel group at the expense of increased bleeding in the prasugrel-treated patients [31]. The dosing regimen of prasugrel for patients with UA/NSTEMI is identical to the dose used in STEMI patients (60 mg load and 10 mg maintenance); it should not be used in patients with a history of stroke or TIA and it should be used with caution in patients over the age of 75 or with a weight less than 60 kg [31].

Ticagrelor, a non-thienopyridine platelet inhibitor that binds reversibly to the P2Y12 platelet receptor, exhibited greater efficacy than clopidogrel in the PLATO trial [70]. Major bleeding events did not differ between the groups, although bleeding not related to coronary artery bypass grafting occurred more often with ticagrelor. Both prasugrel and ticagrelor may have a quicker onset of action than clopidogrel and may prove to be very useful in patients who are clopidogrel-resistant or have recurrent cardiovascular events while on clopidogrel.

The current guidelines recommend a loading dose of 300–600 mg of clopidogrel in patients with UA/NSTEMI followed by 75 mg daily. Prasugrel should be administered as a 60 mg loading dose followed by a 10 mg a day maintenance dose [10]. The duration of clopidogrel may depend on whether or not the patient has received a stent.

Typically patients who received BMSs for at least 4 weeks, and those with DESs should remain on clopidogrel for at least 12 months [9, 10]. For DES, however, adequate long-term data have not been sufficient to formulate a definite recommendation on the duration of therapy.

## Anticoagulant Therapy

Heparin is an important component of primary therapy for patients with unstable coronary syndromes without ST elevation. When added to aspirin, heparin has been shown to reduce refractory angina and the development of myocardial infarction [28], and a meta-analysis of the available data indicates that addition of heparin reduces the composite end point of death or MI [71].

Heparin, however, can be difficult to administer, because the anticoagulant effect is unpredictable in individual patients; this is due to heparin's binding to heparin-binding proteins, endothelial and other cells, and heparin inhibition by several factors released by activated platelets. Therefore, the activated partial thromboplastin time (APTT) must be monitored closely. The potential for heparin-associated thrombocytopenia is also a safety concern.

LMWHs, which are obtained by depolymerization of standard heparin and selection of fractions with lower molecular weight, have several advantages. Because they bind less avidly to heparin-binding proteins, there is less variability in the anticoagulant response and a more predictable dose–response curve, obviating the need to monitor APTT. The incidence of thrombocytopenia is lower (but not absent, and patients with heparin-induced thrombocytopenia with anti-heparin antibodies cannot be switched to LMWH). Finally, LMWHs have longer half-lives, and can be given by subcutaneous injection. These properties make treatment with LMWH at home after hospital discharge feasible. Since evidence suggests that patients with unstable coronary syndromes may remain in a hypercoagulable state for weeks or months, the longer duration of anticoagulation possible with LMWH may be desirable.

Several trials have documented beneficial effects of LMWH therapy in unstable coronary syndromes. The ESSENCE and TIMI 11B trials showed that the LMWH enoxaparin reduced the combined endpoint of death, MI, or recurrent ischemia compared to UFH [72, 73]. The SYNERGY trial found no difference in efficacy between enoxaparin and UFH in high-risk patients, with a slightly higher major bleeding rate [74]. Although LMWH are substantially easier to administer than standard heparin, and long-term administration can be contemplated, they are also more expensive. Specific considerations with the use of LMWH include decreased clearance in renal insufficiency and the lack of a commercially available test to measure the anticoagulant effect. LMWH should be given strong consideration in high-risk patients, but whether substitution of LMWH for heparin in all patients is cost-effective is uncertain.

**Direct Thrombin Inhibitors**

Bivalirudin is a direct thrombin inhibitor, that, unlike heparin, binds directly to both circulating and clot bound thrombin and inhibits the conversion of fibrinogen to fibrin. Direct thrombin inhibitors have several theoretical advantages over heparin, including lack of binding to plasma proteins and lack of binding to platelet factor 4, which avoids the problem of heparin-induced thrombocytopenia.

The REPLACE 2 trial compared bivalirudin plus provisional glycoprotein IIb/IIIa inhibitor to UFH plus planned glycoprotein IIb/IIIa inhibitor in 6,010 patients undergoing planned or urgent PCI, and although 6-month event rates with bivalirudin were slightly higher, bleeding was lower and the prespecified composite endpoint met statistical criteria for non-inferiority [41]. Similar findings were seen in the ACUITY trial, which compared heparin with glycoprotein IIb/IIIa inhibition to bivalirudin with glycoprotein IIb/IIIa inhibition to bivalirudin alone with provisional glycoprotein IIb/IIIa inhibition [37]. Bivalirudin alone compared with heparin plus GP IIb/IIIa inhibitors resulted in noninferior rates of composite ischemia, and reduced major bleeding, but patients who got bivalirudin alone without a thienopyridine prior to angiograpy or PCI had a higher rate of ischemic events. Bilvalirudin should not be administered alone, particularly if there is going to be a delay to angiography.

## *Glycoprotein IIb/IIIa Antagonists*

The benefits of glycoprotein IIb/IIIa inhibitors as adjunctive treatment in patients with ACS have been shown in several trials, with a relative risk reduction of 11% in NSTEMI by meta-analysis [33]. Additional analysis suggests that glycoprotein IIb/IIIa inhibition is most effective in high-risk patients, those with either ECG changes or elevated troponin [33]. The benefits appear to be restricted to patients undergoing percutaneous intervention, which may not be entirely surprising.

These studies were conducted prior to the era of dual antiplatelet therapy. As mentioned previously, it is common practice to administer a thienopyridine and aspirin in conjunction with an anticoagulant in patients with ACS. For patients with UA/NSTEMI undergoing an initial invasive approach, the most recent data suggests that either a glycoprotein IIb/IIIa inhibitor or a thienopyridine can be given in addition to aspirin and an anticoagulant if the patient is considered low risk (troponin negative). However, if the patient is considered high-risk (troponin positive, recurrent ischemic features) both a glycoprotein IIb/IIIa inhibitor and clopidogrel can be given in addition to aspirin and an anticoagulant [9, 10].

## *Interventional Management*

Cardiac catheterization may be undertaken in patients presenting with symptoms suggestive of unstable coronary syndromes for one of several reasons: to assist with risk stratification, as a prelude to revascularization, and to exclude significant epicardial coronary stenosis as a cause of symptoms when the diagnosis is uncertain.

An early invasive approach has now been compared to a conservative approach in several prospective studies. Two earlier trials, the TIMI IIIb study [75] and the VANQWISH trial [76], were negative, but the difference in the number of patients who had been revascularized by the end of these trials was small. In addition, these trials were performed before widespread use of coronary stenting and platelet glycoprotein IIb/IIIa inhibitors, both of which have now been shown to improve outcomes after angioplasty.

The FRISC II, TACTICS-TIMI 18, and RITA III trials each demonstrated that the composite endpoint of death, MI, or refractory angina was less frequent among patients who were randomized to the early invasive strategy, with the greatest benefit observed in high-risk patients: those with elevated cardiac biomarkers, extensive ST segment depression, and hemodynamic features suggestive of large infarctions [77–79].

The ICTUS trial enrolled 1,200 patients with UA/NSTEMI who were initially treated with aspirin and enoxaparin before randomized assignment to one of two strategies: an early invasive strategy within 48 h that included abciximab for PCI or a selective invasive strategy [80]. Patients who were assigned the latter strategy were selected for coronary angiography only if they had refractory angina despite medical treatment, hemodynamic or rhythm instability, or predischarge exercise testing demonstrated clinically significant ischemia. The trial showed no reduction in the composite endpoints of death, nonfatal MI, or rehospitalization for angina at 1 year among patients who were assigned to the early invasive strategy. After 4 years of follow-up, the rates of death and MI among the two groups of patients remained similar [80]. It is not clear why the results of ICTUS differ from previous trials. The more recent timing of intervention in acute coronary syndromes (TIMACS) study randomized 3,031 patients with UA/NSTEMI to undergo cardiac catheterization either within 24 h of symptom onset or more than 36 h later [81]. The median time to angiography was 14 h for the early intervention group and 50 h for the delayed-intervention group. There was no difference between the groups in the composite endpoint of death, myocardial infarction, or stroke at 6 months.

Risk stratification is the key to managing patients with NSTEMI ACS. One possible algorithm for managing patients with NSTEMI is shown in Fig. 2.2. An initial strategy of medical management with attempts at stabilization is warranted in patients with lower risk, but patients at higher risk should be considered for cardiac catheterization. Pharmacologic and mechanical strategies are intertwined in the sense that selection of patients for early revascularization will influence the choice of antiplatelet and anticoagulant medication. When good clinical judgment is employed, early coronary angiography in selected patients with ACS can lead to better management and lower morbidity and mortality.

It is important to be aware that if a fibrinolytic agent was chosen as a means of reperfusion in ST-segment elevation MI, success is by no means guaranteed. Should the patient continue to show clinical signs (ongoing chest pain, hemodynamic or electrical instability) or ECG evidence (failure of resolution of ST-segment elevation by >50%) of ongoing cardiac ischemia, immediate transfer to a PCI capable site

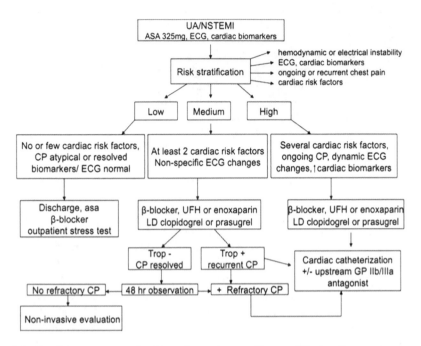

**Fig. 2.2** Possible treatment algorithm for patients with non-ST elevation acute coronary syndromes. *ASA* aspirin; *CP* chest pain; *ECG* electrocardiogram; *GPIIb/IIIa* glycoprotein IIb/IIIa antagonist; *LD* loading dose; *Trop* troponin; *UFH* unfractionated heparin

should be initiated. In an effort to address the question of how to best handle the possibility of failed fibrinolysis, and when exactly to perform cardiac catheterization and PCI, the TRANSFER-AMI study randomized 1,059 high-risk patients with STEMI given fibrinolytic therapy at centers without PCI capability to immediate transfer to a PCI capable institution vs. usual care [82]. The trial demonstrated benefit with early PCI following thrombolytic therapy for ST-segment elevation MI, regardless of whether lytic therapy was effective in reperfusion. This strategy, termed "pharmacoinvasive," resulted in a decrease in the primary endpoint of death, MI, heart failure, severe recurrent ischemia, or shock by 6.2% (11.0 vs. 17.2%) as well as secondary endpoints of reinfarction and recurrent ischemia when compared to patients receiving standard treatment [82].

## Complications of Acute Myocardial Infarction

### Postinfarction Ischemia

Causes of ischemia after infarction include decreased myocardial oxygen supply due to coronary reocclusion or spasm, mechanical problems that increase myocardial oxygen demand, and extracardiac factors such as hypertension, anemia, hypotension, or hypermetabolic states. Nonischemic causes of chest pain, such as postinfarction pericarditis and acute pulmonary embolism, should also be considered.

Immediate management includes aspirin, β-blockade, IV nitroglycerin, heparin, and diagnostic coronary angiography. Post-infarction angina is an indication for revascularization. PTCA can be performed if the culprit lesion is suitable. CABG should be considered for patients with left main disease, three-vessel disease, and those unsuitable for PTCA. If the angina cannot be controlled medically or is accompanied by hemodynamic instability, an intra-aortic balloon pump should be inserted.

## Ventricular Free Wall Rupture

Ventricular free wall rupture typically occurs during the first week after infarction. The classic patient is elderly, female, and hypertensive. Early use of thrombolytic therapy reduces the incidence of cardiac rupture, but late use may actually increase the risk. Pseudoaneursym with leakage may be heralded by chest pain, nausea, and restlessness, but frank free wall rupture presents as a catastrophic event with shock and electromechanical dissociation. Pericardiocentesis may be necessary to relieve acute tamponade, ideally in the operating room, since the pericardial effusion may be tamponading the bleeding. Salvage is possible with prompt recognition, pericardiocentesis to relieve acute tamponade, and thoracotomy with repair [83]. A pericardial effusion may be seen by echocardiography: contrast ventriculography is not a sensitive way to detect a small rupture.

## Ventricular Septal Rupture

Septal rupture presents as severe heart failure or cardiogenic shock, with a pansystolic murmur and parasternal thrill. The hallmark finding is a left-to-right intracardiac shunt ("step-up" in oxygen saturation from right atrium to right ventricle), but the diagnosis is most easily made with echocardiography.

Rapid institution of intra-aortic balloon pumping and supportive pharmacologic measures is necessary. Operative repair is the only viable option for long-term survival. The timing of surgery has been controversial, but most authorities now suggest that repair should be undertaken early, within 48 h of the rupture [84].

## Acute Mitral Regurgitation

Ischemic mitral regurgitation is usually associated with inferior myocardial infarction and ischemia or infarction of the posterior papillary muscle, although anterior papillary muscle rupture can also occur. Papillary muscle rupture has a bimodal incidence, either within 24 h or 3–7 days after acute myocardial infarction, and usually presents dramatically, with pulmonary edema, hypotension, and cardiogenic shock. When a papillary muscle ruptures, the murmur of acute mitral regurgitation may be limited to early systole because of rapid equalization of pressures in the left atrium and left ventricle. More importantly, the murmur may be soft or inaudible, especially when cardiac output is low [85].

Echocardiography is extremely useful in the differential diagnosis, which includes free wall rupture, ventricular septal rupture, and infarct extension with pump failure. Hemodynamic monitoring with pulmonary artery catheterization may also be helpful. Management includes afterload reduction with nitroprusside and intra-aortic balloon pumping as temporizing measures. Inotropic or vasopressor therapy may also be needed to support cardiac output and blood pressure. Definitive therapy, however, is surgical valve repair or replacement, which should be undertaken as soon as possible since clinical deterioration can be sudden [85–87].

## Right Ventricular Infarction

Right ventricular infarction occurs in up to 30% of patients with inferior infarction and is clinically significant in 10% [88]. The combination of a clear chest X-ray with jugular venous distention in a patient with an inferior wall MI should lead to the suspicion of a coexisting right ventricular infarct. The diagnosis is substantiated by demonstration of ST segment elevation in the right precordial leads ($V_{3R}$–$V_{5R}$) or by characteristic hemodynamic findings on right heart catheterization (elevated right atrial and right ventricular end-diastolic pressures with normal to low pulmonary artery occlusion pressure and low cardiac output). Echocardiography can demonstrate depressed right ventricular contractility [89]. Patients with cardiogenic shock on the basis of right ventricular infarction have a better prognosis than those with left-sided pump failure [88]. This may be due in part to the fact that right ventricular function tends to return to normal over time with supportive therapy [90], although such therapy may need to be prolonged.

In patients with right ventricular infarction, right ventricular preload should be maintained with fluid administration. In some cases, however, fluid resuscitation may increase pulmonary capillary occlusion pressure but may not increase cardiac output, and overdilation of the right ventricle can compromise left ventricular filling and cardiac output [90]. Inotropic therapy with dobutamine may be more effective in increasing cardiac output in some patients, and monitoring with serial echocardiograms may also be useful to detect right ventricular overdistention [90]. Maintenance of atrioventricular synchrony is also important in these patients to optimize right ventricular filling [89]. For patients with continued hemodynamic instability, intra-aortic balloon pumping may be useful, particularly because elevated right ventricular pressures and volumes increase wall stress and oxygen consumption and decrease right coronary perfusion pressure, exacerbating right ventricular ischemia.

Reperfusion of the occluded coronary artery is also crucial. A study using direct angioplasty demonstrated that restoration of normal flow resulted in dramatic recovery of right ventricular function and a mortality rate of only 2%, whereas unsuccessful reperfusion was associated with persistent hemodynamic compromise and a mortality of 58% [91].

## Cardiogenic Shock

### Epidemiology and Pathophysiology

Cardiogenic shock, resulting either from left ventricular pump failure or from mechanical complications, represents the leading cause of in-hospital death after myocardial infarction [92]. Despite advances in management of heart failure and acute myocardial infarction, until very recently, clinical outcomes in patients with cardiogenic shock have been poor, with reported mortality rates ranging from 50 to 80% [93]. Patients may have cardiogenic shock at initial presentation, but shock often evolves over several hours [94, 95].

Cardiac dysfunction in patients with cardiogenic shock is usually initiated by myocardial infarction or ischemia. The myocardial dysfunction resulting from ischemia worsens that ischemia, creating a downward spiral (Fig. 2.3). Compensatory mechanisms that retain fluid in an attempt to maintain cardiac output may add to the vicious cycle and further increase diastolic filling pressures. The interruption of this cycle of myocardial dysfunction and ischemia forms the basis for the therapeutic regimens for cardiogenic shock.

Initial Management

Maintenance of adequate oxygenation and ventilation are critical. Many patients require intubation and mechanical ventilation, if only to reduce the work of breathing and facilitate sedation and stabilization before cardiac catheterization. Electrolyte abnormalities should be corrected, and morphine used to relieve pain and anxiety, thus reducing excessive sympathetic activity and decreasing oxygen demand, preload, and afterload. Arrhythmias and heart block may have major effects on cardiac output, and should be corrected promptly with antiarrhythmic drugs, cardioversion, or pacing.

The initial approach to the hypotensive patient should include fluid resuscitation unless frank pulmonary edema is present. Patients are commonly diaphoretic and relative hypovolemia may be present in as many as 20% of patients with cardiogenic shock. Fluid infusion is best initiated with predetermined boluses titrated to clinical endpoints of heart rate, urine output and blood pressure. Ischemia produces diastolic as well as systolic dysfunction, and thus elevated filling pressures may be necessary to maintain stroke volume in patients with cardiogenic shock. Patients who do not respond rapidly to initial fluid boluses or those with poor physiologic

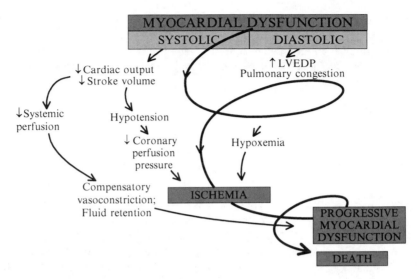

**Fig. 2.3** The "downward spiral" in cardiogenic shock. Stroke volume and cardiac output fall with left ventricular (LV) dysfunction, producing hypotension and tachycardia that reduce coronary blood flow. Increasing ventricular diastolic pressure reduces coronary blood flow, and increased wall stress elevates myocardial oxygen requirements. All of these factors combine to worsen ischemia. The falling cardiac output also compromises systemic perfusion. Compensatory mechanisms include sympathetic stimulation and fluid retention to increase preload. These mechanisms can actually worsen cardiogenic shock by increasing myocardial oxygen demand and afterload. Thus, a vicious circle can be established. LVEDP, left ventricular end-diastolic pressure. Adapted with permission from Hollenberg et al. [92]

reserve should be considered for invasive hemodynamic monitoring. Optimal filling pressures vary from patient to patient; hemodynamic monitoring can be used to construct a Starling curve at the bedside, identifying the filling pressure at which cardiac output is maximized. Maintenance of adequate preload is particularly important in patients with right ventricular infarction.

When arterial pressure remains inadequate, therapy with vasopressor agents may be required to maintain coronary perfusion pressure. Maintenance of adequate blood pressure is essential to break the vicious cycle of progressive hypotension with further myocardial ischemia. Dopamine increases both blood pressure and cardiac output, but recent data suggest that norepinephrine may be a superior agent in patients with cardiogenic shock [96]. Phenylephrine, a selective alpha-1 adrenergic agonist, may be useful when tachyarrhythmias limit therapy with other vasopressors. Vasopressor infusions need to be titrated carefully in patients with cardiogenic shock to maximize coronary perfusion pressure with the least possible increase in myocardial oxygen demand. Hemodynamic monitoring, with serial measurements of cardiac output, filling pressures (and other parameters, such as mixed venous oxygen saturation) allows for titration of the dosage of vasoactive agents to the minimum dosage required to achieve the chosen therapeutic goals [97].

Following initial stabilization and restoration of adequate blood pressure, tissue perfusion should be assessed. If tissue perfusion remains inadequate, inotropic support or intra-aortic balloon pumping should be initiated. If tissue perfusion is adequate but significant pulmonary congestion remains, diuretics may be employed. Vasodilators can be considered as well, depending on the blood pressure.

In patients with inadequate tissue perfusion and adequate intravascular volume, cardiovascular support with inotropic agents should be initiated. Dobutamine, a selective β1-adrenergic receptor agonist, can improve myocardial contractility and increase cardiac output, and is the initial agent of choice in patients with systolic pressures greater than 80 mmHg. Dobutamine may exacerbate hypotension in some patients, and can precipitate tachyarrhythmias. Use of dopamine may be preferable if systolic pressure is less than 80 mmHg, although tachycardia and increased peripheral resistance may worsen myocardial ischemia. Phosphodiesterase inhibitors such as milrinone are less arrhythmogenic than catecholamines, but have the potential to cause hypotension, and should be used with caution in patients with tenuous clinical status. Levosimendan, a calcium sensitizer, has both inotropic and vasodilator properties and does not increase myocardial oxygen consumption. Several relatively small studies have shown hemodynamic benefits with levosimendan in cardiogenic shock after MI [98, 99], but survival benefits have not been shown either in cardiogenic shock or acute heart failure [100].

Intra-aortic balloon counterpulsation (IABP) reduces systolic afterload and augments diastolic perfusion pressure, increasing cardiac output and improving coronary blood flow [101]. These beneficial effects, in contrast to those of inotropic or vasopressor agents, occur without an increase in oxygen demand. IABP does not, however, produce a significant improvement in blood flow distal to a critical coronary stenosis, and has not been shown to improve mortality when used alone without reperfusion therapy or revascularization. In patients with cardiogenic shock and compromised tissue perfusion, IABP can be an essential support mechanism to stabilize patients and allow time for definitive therapeutic measures to be undertaken [101, 102]. In appropriate settings, more intensive support with mechanical assist devices may also be implemented.

## Reperfusion Therapy

Although thrombolytic therapy reduces the likelihood of subsequent development of shock after initial presentation [95], its role in the management of patients who have already developed shock is less certain. The available randomized trials have not demonstrated that fibrinolytic therapy reduces mortality in patients with established cardiogenic shock. On the other hand, in the SHOCK Registry, patients treated with fibrinolytic therapy had a lower in-hospital mortality rate than those who were not (54 vs. 64%, $p = 0.005$), even after adjustment for age and revascularization status (OR 0.70, $p = 0.027$) [103].

Fibrinolytic therapy is clearly less effective in patients with cardiogenic shock than in those without. The explanation for this lack of efficacy appears to be the low reperfusion rate achieved in this subset of patients. The reasons for decreased thrombolytic efficacy in patients with cardiogenic shock probably include hemodynamic, mechanical, and metabolic factors that prevent achievement and maintenance of infarct-related artery patency [104]. Attempts to increase reperfusion rates by increasing blood pressure with aggressive inotropic and pressor therapy and IABP make theoretic sense, and two small studies support the notion that vasopressor therapy to increase aortic pressure improves thrombolytic efficacy [104, 105]. The use of intra-aortic balloon pumping to augment aortic diastolic pressure may increase the effectiveness of thrombolytics as well.

To date, emergency percutaneous revascularization is the only intervention that has been shown to consistently reduce mortality rates in patients with cardiogenic shock. An extensive body of observational and registry studies has shown consistent benefits from revascularization but could not be regarded as definitive due to their retrospective design. These data have now been supported by randomized controlled trials.

The SHOCK study was a randomized, multicenter international trial that assigned patients with cardiogenic shock to receive optimal medical management – including IABP and thrombolytic therapy – or to cardiac catheterization with revascularization using PTCA or CABG [106, 107]. The primary endpoint, all-cause mortality at 30 days, was 46.7% in the revascularization group, and 56% in the medical therapy group, a difference that did not reach statistical significance ($p = 0.11$) [107]. Planned follow-up, however, revealed a significant benefit from early revascularization at 6 months and at 1 year ($p < 0.03$) [107]. Subgroup analyses also revealed benefit in patients younger than 75 years, those with prior MI, and those randomized less than 6 h from onset of infarction [106, 107].

The SMASH trial was similarly designed, but enrolled sicker patients [108]. The trial was terminated early due to difficulties in patient recruitment, and enrolled only 55 patients, but a reduction in 30-day absolute mortality reduction similar to that in the SHOCK trial (69% mortality in the invasive group vs. 78% in the medically managed group, $p = NS$) [108], and this benefit was also maintained at 1 year.

When the results of both the SHOCK and SMASH trials are put into perspective with results from other randomized, controlled trials of patients with acute myocardial infarction, an important point emerges: despite the moderate relative risk reduction (for the SHOCK trial: 0.72, CI 0.54–0.95; for the SMASH trial: 0.88, CI 0.60–1.20) the absolute benefit is important, with 9 lives saved for 100 patients treated at 30 days in both trials, and 13.2 lives saved for 100 patients treated at 1 year in the SHOCK trial. This latter figure corresponds to a number needed to treat (NNT) of 7.6, one of the lowest figures observed in a randomized, controlled trial of cardiovascular disease.

On the basis of these randomized trials, the presence of cardiogenic shock in the setting of acute MI is a class I indication for emergency revascularization, either by percutaneous intervention or CABG [10].

# References

1. Libby P. Current concepts of the pathogenesis of the acute coronary syndromes. Circulation. 2001;104:365-72.
2. Ambrose JA, Martinez EE. A new paradigm for plaque stabilization. Circulation. 2002;105:2000-4.
3. Croft CH, Nicod P, Corbett JR, et al. Detection of acute right ventricular infarction by right precordial electrocardiography. Am J Cardiol. 1982;50:421-7.
4. Spodick DH. Diagnostic electrocardiographic sequences in acute pericarditis. Significance of PR segment and PR vector changes. Circulation. 1973;48:575-80.
5. Goodman SG, Fu Y, Langer A, et al. The prognostic value of the admission and predischarge electrocardiogram in acute coronary syndromes: the GUSTO-IIb ECG Core Laboratory experience. Am Heart J. 2006;152:277-84.
6. Zimmerman J, Fromm R, Meyer D, et al. Diagnostic marker cooperative study for the diagnosis of myocardial infarction. Circulation. 1999;99:1671-7.
7. Saenger AK, Jaffe AS. Requiem for a heavyweight: the demise of creatine kinase-MB. Circulation. 2008;118:2200-6.
8. Jaffe AS, Babuin L, Apple FS. Biomarkers in acute cardiac disease: the present and the future. J Am Coll Cardiol. 2006;48:1-11.
9. Anderson JL, Adams CD, Antman EM, et al. ACC/AHA 2007 guidelines for the management of patients with unstable angina/non ST-elevation myocardial infarction: a report of the American College of Cardiology/American Heart Association Task Force on Practice Guidelines. Circulation. 2007;106:803-77.
10. Kushner FG, Hand M, Smith Jr SC, et al. 2009 Focused updates: ACC/AHA Guidelines for the Management of Patients With ST-Elevation Myocardial Infarction (updating the 2004 Guideline and 2007 Focused Update) and ACC/AHA/SCAI Guidelines on Percutaneous Coronary Intervention (updating the 2005 Guideline and 2007 Focused Update): a report of the American College of Cardiology Foundation/American Heart Association Task Force on Practice Guidelines. Circulation. 2009;120:2271-330.
11. Gruppo Italiano per lo Studio Della Streptochinasi Nell'Infarto Miocardico (GISSI). Effectiveness of intravenous thrombolytic treatment in acute myocardial infarction. Lancet. 1986;2:397-402.
12. TIMI Study Group. The thrombolysis in myocardial infarction (TIMI) trial. Phase I findings. N Engl J Med. 1985;312:932-6.
13. GUSTO Angiographic Investigators. The effects of tissue plasminogen activator, streptokinase, or both on coronary-artery patency, ventricular function, and survival after acute myocardial infarction. N Engl J Med. 1993;329:1615-22.
14. GUSTO Investigators. An international randomized trial comparing four thrombolytic strategies for acute myocardial infarction. N Engl J Med. 1993;329:673-82.
15. Global Use of Strategies to Open Occluded Coronary Arteries (GUSTO III) Investigators. A comparison of reteplase with alteplase for acute myocardial infarction. N Engl J Med. 1997;337:1118-23.
16. Assessment of the Safety and Efficacy of a New Thrombolytic Investigators. Single-bolus tenecteplase compared with front-loaded alteplase in acute myocardial infarction: the ASSENT-2 double-blind randomised trial. Lancet. 1999;354:716-22.
17. Grines CL, Browne KF, Marco J, et al. A comparison of immediate angioplasty with thrombolytic therapy for acute myocardial infarction. N Engl J Med. 1993;328:673-9.
18. GUSTO IIb Investigators. A comparison of recombinant hirudin with heparin for the treatment of acute coronary syndromes. N Engl J Med. 1996;335:775-82.
19. Grines C, Patel A, Zijlstra F, Weaver WD, Granger C, Simes RJ. Primary coronary angioplasty compared with intravenous thrombolytic therapy for acute myocardial infarction: six-month follow up and analysis of individual patient data from randomized trials. Am Heart J. 2003;145:47-57.

20. Keeley EC, Boura JA, Grines CL. Primary angioplasty versus intravenous thrombolytic therapy for acute myocardial infarction: a quantitative review of 23 randomised trials. Lancet. 2003;361:13–20.
21. Cannon CP, Gibson CM, Lambrew CT, et al. Relationship of symptom-onset-to-balloon time and door-to-balloon time with mortality in patients undergoing angioplasty for acute myocardial infarction. JAMA. 2000;283:2941–7.
22. Anderson RD, White HD, Ohman EM, et al. Predicting outcome after thrombolysis in acute myocardial infarction according to ST-segment resolution at 90 minutes: a substudy of the GUSTO III trial. Am Heart J. 2002;144:81–8.
23. Schroder R, Dissmann R, Bruggemann T, et al. Extent of early ST segment elevation resolution: a simple but strong predictor of outcome in patients with acute myocardial infarction. J Am Coll Cardiol. 1994;24:384–91.
24. Rankin JM, Spinelli JJ, Carere RG, et al. Improved clinical outcome after widespread use of coronary-artery stenting in Canada. N Engl J Med. 1999;341:1957–65.
25. Stone GW, Brodie BR, Griffin JJ, et al. Clinical and angiographic follow-up after primary stenting in acute myocardial infarction: the Primary Angioplasty in Myocardial Infarction (PAMI) stent pilot trial. Circulation. 1999;99:1548–54.
26. ISIS-2 Collaborative Group. Randomised trial of intravenous streptokinase, oral aspirin, both, or neither among 17 187 cases of suspected acute myocardial infarction: ISIS-2. Lancet. 1988;2:349–60.
27. Lewis Jr HD, Davis JW, Archibald DG, et al. Protective effects of aspirin against acute myocardial infarction and death in men with unstable angina. Results of a Veterans Administration Cooperative Study. N Engl J Med. 1983;309:396–403.
28. Theroux P, Ouimet H, McCans J, et al. Aspirin, heparin, or both to treat acute unstable angina. N Engl J Med. 1988;319:1105–11.
29. Sabatine MS, Cannon CP, Gibson CM, et al. Addition of clopidogrel to aspirin and fibrinolytic therapy for myocardial infarction with ST-segment elevation. N Engl J Med. 2005;352:1179–89.
30. Sabatine MS, Cannon CP, Gibson CM, et al. Effect of clopidogrel pretreatment before percutaneous coronary intervention in patients with ST-elevation myocardial infarction treated with fibrinolytics: the PCI-CLARITY study. JAMA. 2005;294:1224–32.
31. Wiviott SD, Braunwald E, McCabe CH, et al. Prasugrel versus clopidogrel in patients with acute coronary syndromes. N Engl J Med. 2007;357:2001–15.
32. Chen ZM, Jiang LX, Chen YP, et al. Addition of clopidogrel to aspirin in 45,852 patients with acute myocardial infarction: randomised placebo-controlled trial. Lancet. 2005;366:1607–21.
33. Chew DP, Moliterno DJ. A critical appraisal of platelet glycoprotein IIb/IIIa inhibition. J Am Coll Cardiol. 2000;36:2028–35.
34. Montalescot G, Barragan P, Wittenberg O, et al. Platelet glycoprotein IIb/IIIa inhibition with coronary stenting for acute myocardial infarction. N Engl J Med. 2001;344:1895–903.
35. Stone GW, Grines CL, Cox DA, et al. Comparison of angioplasty with stenting, with or without abciximab, in acute myocardial infarction. N Engl J Med. 2002;346:957–66.
36. Mehilli J, Kastrati A, Schulz S, et al. Abciximab in patients with acute ST-segment-elevation myocardial infarction undergoing primary percutaneous coronary intervention after clopidogrel loading: a randomized double-blind trial. Circulation. 2009;119:1933–40.
37. Stone GW, Witzenbichler B, Guagliumi G, et al. Bivalirudin during primary PCI in acute myocardial infarction. N Engl J Med. 2008;358:2218–30.
38. Van't Hof AW, Ten Berg J, Heestermans T. Prehospital initiation of tirofiban in patients with ST-elevation myocardial infarction undergoing primary angioplasty (On-TIME 2): a multicentre, double-blind, randomised controlled trial. Lancet. 2008;372:537–46.
39. Antman EM, Morrow DA, McCabe CH, et al. Enoxaparin versus unfractionated heparin with fibrinolysis for ST-elevation myocardial infarction. N Engl J Med. 2006;354:1477–88.
40. Wallentin L, Goldstein P, Armstrong PW, et al. Efficacy and safety of tenecteplase in combination with the low-molecular-weight heparin enoxaparin or unfractionated heparin in the

prehospital setting: the Assessment of the Safety and Efficacy of a New Thrombolytic Regimen (ASSENT)-3 PLUS randomized trial in acute myocardial infarction. Circulation. 2003;108:135–42.

41. Lincoff AM, Bittl JA, Harrington RA, et al. Bivalirudin and provisional glycoprotein IIb/IIIa blockade compared with heparin and planned glycoprotein IIb/IIIa blockade during percutaneous coronary intervention: REPLACE-2 randomized trial. JAMA. 2003;289:853–63.

42. Mehran R, Brodie B, Cox DA, et al. The Harmonizing Outcomes with RevasculariZatiON and Stents in Acute Myocardial Infarction (HORIZONS-AMI) Trial: study design and rationale. Am Heart J. 2008;156:44–56.

43. Cohn PF, Gorlin R. Physiologic and clinical actions of nitroglycerin. Med Clin North Am. 1974;58:407–15.

44. Gruppo Italiano per lo Studio Della Sopravvinza Nell'Infarto Miocardico (GISSI). GISSI-3: effects of lisinopril and transdermal glyceryl trinitrate singly and together on 6-week mortality and ventricular function after acute myocardial infarction. Lancet. 1994;343:1115–22.

45. ISIS-4 (Fourth International Study of Infarct Survival) Study Group. ISIS-4: a randomised factorial trial assessing early oral captopril, oral mononitrate, and intravenous magnesium sulphate in 58,050 patients with suspected acute myocardial infarction. Lancet. 1995;345: 669–85.

46. First International Study of Infarct Survival Collaborative Group. Randomised trial of intravenous atenolol among 16 027 cases of suspected acute myocardial infarction: ISIS-1. Lancet. 1986;2:57–66.

47. TIMI Study Group. Comparison of invasive and conservative strategies after treatment with intravenous tissue plasminogen activator in acute myocardial infarction. Results of the Thrombolysis in Myocardial Infarction (TIMI) Phase II Trial. N Engl J Med. 1989;320: 618–27.

48. Chen ZM, Pan HC, Chen YP, et al. Early intravenous then oral metoprolol in 45,852 patients with acute myocardial infarction: randomised placebo-controlled trial. Lancet. 2005;366:1622–32.

49. MIAMI Trial Research Group. Metoprolol in acute myocardial infarction (MIAMI). A randomised placebo-controlled international trial. Eur Heart J. 1985;6:199–226.

50. Dargie HJ. Effect of carvedilol on outcome after myocardial infarction in patients with left-ventricular dysfunction: the CAPRICORN randomised trial. Lancet. 2001;357:1385–90.

51. Lipid Research Clinics Program. The lipid research clinics coronary primary prevention trial results. II. The relationship of reduction in incidence of coronary heart disease to cholesterol lowering. JAMA. 1984;251:365–74.

52. Frick MH, Elo O, Haapa K, et al. Helsinki heart study: primary-prevention trial with gemfibrozil in middle-aged men with dyslipidemia. Safety of treatment, changes in risk factors, and incidence of coronary heart disease. N Engl J Med. 1987;317:1237–45.

53. Heart Protection Study Collaborative Group. MRC/BHF Heart Protection Study of cholesterol lowering with simvastatin in 20,536 high-risk individuals: a randomised placebo-controlled trial. Lancet. 2002;360:7–22.

54. Ridker PM, Danielson E, Fonseca FA, et al. Rosuvastatin to prevent vascular events in men and women with elevated C-reactive protein. N Engl J Med. 2008;359:2195–207.

55. Long-Term Intervention with Pravastatin in Ischaemic Disease (LIPID) Study Group. Prevention of cardiovascular events and death with pravastatin in patients with coronary heart disease and a broad range of initial cholesterol levels. N Engl J Med. 1998;339:1349–57.

56. Sacks FM, Pfeffer MA, Moye LA, et al. The effect of pravastatin on coronary events after myocardial infarction in patients with average cholesterol levels. N Engl J Med. 1996;335: 1001–9.

57. Scandinavian Simvastatin Survival Study Group. Randomised trial of cholesterol lowering in 4444 patients with coronary heart disease: the Scandinavian Simvastatin Survival Study (4S). Lancet. 1994;344:1383–9.

58. Gibbons RJ, Abrams J, Chatterjee K, et al. ACC/AHA 2002 guideline update for the management of patients with chronic stable angina – summary article: a report of the American College of Cardiology/American Heart Association Task Force on Practice Guidelines

(Committee on the Management of Patients With Chronic Stable Angina). Circulation. 2003;107:149–58.

59. Grundy SM, Cleeman JI, Merz CN, et al. Implications of recent clinical trials for the National Cholesterol Education Program Adult Treatment Panel III guidelines. Circulation. 2004;110: 227–39.

60. Pfeffer MA, Braunwald E, Moye LA, et al. Effect of captopril on mortality and morbidity in patients with left ventricular dysfunction after myocardial infarction. Results of the Survival and Ventricular Enlargement Trial. N Engl J Med. 1992;327:669–77.

61. Swedberg K, Held P, Kjekshus J, et al. Effects of the early administration of enalapril on mortality in patients with acute myocardial infarction. Results of the Cooperative New Scandinavian Enalapril Survival Study II (CONSENSUS II). N Engl J Med. 1992;327: 678–84.

62. Furberg CD, Psaty BM, Meyer JV. Nifedipine. Dose-related increase in mortality in patients with coronary heart disease. Circulation. 1995;92:1326–31.

63. Gibson RS, Boden WE, Theroux P, et al. Diltiazem and reinfarction in patients with non-q-wave myocardial infarction. N Engl J Med. 1986;315:423–9.

64. MacMahon S, Collins R, Peto R, Koster RW, Yusuf S. Effects of prophylactic lidocaine in suspected acute myocardial infarction. An overview of results from the randomized, controlled trials. J Am Med Assoc. 1988;260:1910–6.

65. Lauler DP. Magnesium – coming of age. Am J Cardiol. 1989;63:1g–3.

66. Braunwald E. Unstable angina. A classification. Circulation. 1989;80:413–4.

67. Ohman EM, Armstrong PW, Christenson RH, et al. Cardiac troponin T levels for risk stratification in acute myocardial ischemia. N Engl J Med. 1996;335:1333–41.

68. Cairns JA, Gent M, Singer J, et al. Aspirin, sulfinpyrazone, or both in unstable angina. Results of a Canadian multicenter trial. N Engl J Med. 1985;313:1369–75.

69. Yusuf S, Zhao F, Mehta SR, Chrolavicius S, Tognoni G, Fox KK. Effects of clopidogrel in addition to aspirin in patients with acute coronary syndromes without ST-segment elevation. N Engl J Med. 2001;345:494–502.

70. Wallentin L, Becker RC, Budaj A, et al. Ticagrelor versus clopidogrel in patients with acute coronary syndromes. N Engl J Med. 2009;361:1045–57.

71. Oler A, Whooley MA, Oler J, Grady D. Adding heparin to aspirin reduces the incidence of myocardial infarction and death in patients with unstable angina. A meta-analysis. JAMA. 1996;276:811–5.

72. Cohen M, Demers C, Gurfinkel EP, et al. A comparison of low-molecular-weight heparin with unfractionated heparin for unstable coronary artery disease. Efficacy and Safety of Subcutaneous Enoxaparin in Non-Q-Wave Coronary Events Study Group. N Engl J Med. 1997;337:447–52.

73. Antman EM, McCabe CH, Gurfinkel EP, et al. Enoxaparin prevents death and cardiac ischemic events in unstable angina/non-Q-wave myocardial infarction. Results of the thrombolysis in myocardial infarction (TIMI) 11B trial. Circulation. 1999;100:1593–601.

74. Ferguson JJ, Califf RM, Antman EM, et al. Enoxaparin vs unfractionated heparin in high-risk patients with non-ST-segment elevation acute coronary syndromes managed with an intended early invasive strategy: primary results of the SYNERGY randomized trial. JAMA. 2004;292:45–54.

75. Investigators TIMI. Effects of tissue plasminogen activator and a comparison of early invasive and conservative strategies in unstable angina and non-Q-wave myocardial infarction. Results of the TIMI IIIB trial. Circulation. 1994;89:1545–56.

76. Boden WE, O'Rourke RA, Crawford MH, et al. Outcomes in patients with acute non-Q-wave myocardial infarction randomly assigned to an invasive as compared with a conservative management strategy. N Engl J Med. 1998;338:1785–92.

77. FRagmin and Fast Revascularisation during InStability in Coronary artery disease Investigators. Invasive compared with non-invasive treatment in unstable coronary-artery disease: FRISC II prospective randomised multicentre study. Lancet. 1999;354:708–15.

78. Cannon CP, Weintraub WS, Demopoulos LA, et al. Comparison of early invasive and conservative strategies in patients with unstable coronary syndromes treated with the glycoprotein IIb/IIIa inhibitor tirofiban. N Engl J Med. 2001;344:1879–87.

79. RITA Trial Participants. Coronary angioplasty versus coronary artery bypass surgery: the Randomised Intervention Treatment of Angina (RITA) trial. Lancet. 1993;341:573–80.

80. Hirsch A, Windhausen F, Tijssen JG, Verheugt FW, Cornel JH, de Winter RJ. Long-term outcome after an early invasive versus selective invasive treatment strategy in patients with non-ST-elevation acute coronary syndrome and elevated cardiac troponin T (the ICTUS trial): a follow-up study. Lancet. 2007;369:827–35.

81. Mehta SR, Granger CB, Boden WE, et al. Early versus delayed invasive intervention in acute coronary syndromes. N Engl J Med. 2009;360:2165–75.

82. Cantor WJ, Fitchett D, Borgundvaag B, et al. Routine early angioplasty after fibrinolysis for acute myocardial infarction. N Engl J Med. 2009;360:2705–18.

83. Reardon MJ, Carr CL, Diamond A, et al. Ischemic left ventricular free wall rupture: prediction, diagnosis, and treatment. Ann Thorac Surg. 1997;64:1509–13.

84. Killen DA, Piehler JM, Borkon AM, Gorton ME, Reed WA. Early repair of postinfarction ventricular septal rupture. Ann Thorac Surg. 1997;63:138–42.

85. Khan SS, Gray RJ. Valvular emergencies. Cardiol Clin. 1991;9:689–709.

86. Bolooki H. Emergency cardiac procedures in patients in cardiogenic shock due to complications of coronary artery disease. Circulation. 1989;79:I137–48.

87. Carabello BA. The current therapy for mitral regurgitation. J Am Coll Cardiol. 2008;52: 319–26.

88. Zehender M, Kasper W, Kauder E, et al. Right ventricular infarction as an independent predictor of prognosis after acute inferior myocardial infarction. N Engl J Med. 1993;328:981–8.

89. Nedeljkovic ZS, Ryan TJ. Right ventricular infarction. In: Hollenberg SM, Bates ER, editors. Cardiogenic shock. Armonk, NY: Futura; 2002. p. 161–86.

90. Dell'Italia LJ, Starling MR, Blumhardt R, Lasher JC, O'Rourke RA. Comparative effects of volume loading, dobutamine, and nitroprusside in patients with predominant right ventricular infarction. Circulation. 1985;72:1327–35.

91. Bowers TR, O'Neill WW, Grines C, Pica MC, Safian RD, Goldstein JA. Effect of reperfusion on biventricular function and survival after right ventricular infarction. N Engl J Med. 1998;338:933–40.

92. Hollenberg SM, Kavinsky CJ, Parrillo JE. Cardiogenic shock. Ann Intern Med. 1999;131: 47–59.

93. Goldberg RJ, Spencer FA, Gore JM, Lessard D, Yarzebski J. Thirty-year trends (1975 to 2005) in the magnitude of, management of, and hospital death rates associated with cardiogenic shock in patients with acute myocardial infarction: a population-based perspective. Circulation. 2009;119:1211–9.

94. Hochman JS, Boland J, Sleeper LA, et al. Current spectrum of cardiogenic shock and effect of early revascularization on mortality. Results of an International Registry. Circulation. 1995;91:873–81.

95. Holmes Jr DR, Bates ER, Kleiman NS, et al. Contemporary reperfusion therapy for cardiogenic shock: the GUSTO-I trial experience. The GUSTO-I Investigators. Global utilization of streptokinase and tissue plasminogen activator for occluded coronary arteries. J Am Coll Cardiol. 1995;26:668–74.

96. De Backer D, Biston P, Devriendt J, et al. Comparison of dopamine and norepinephrine in the treatment of shock. N Engl J Med. 2010;362:779–89.

97. Hollenberg SM, Parrillo JE. Shock. In: Fauci AS, Braunwald E, Isselbacher KJ, et al., editors. Harrison's principles of internal medicine. 14th ed. New York: McGraw-Hill; 1997. p. 214–22.

98. Garcia-Gonzalez MJ, Dominguez-Rodriguez A, Ferrer-Hita JJ, Abreu-Gonzalez P, Munoz MB. Cardiogenic shock after primary percutaneous coronary intervention: effects of levosimendan compared with dobutamine on haemodynamics. Eur J Heart Fail. 2006;8:723–8.

99. Russ MA, Prondzinsky R, Christoph A, et al. Hemodynamic improvement following levosimendan treatment in patients with acute myocardial infarction and cardiogenic shock. Crit Care Med. 2007;35:2732–9.

100. Mebazaa A, Nieminen MS, Packer M, et al. Levosimendan vs dobutamine for patients with acute decompensated heart failure: the SURVIVE randomized trial. JAMA. 2007;297:1883–91.

101. Willerson JT, Curry GC, Watson JT, et al. Intraaortic balloon counterpulsation in patients in cardiogenic shock, medically refractory left ventricular failure and/or recurrent ventricular tachycardia. Am J Med. 1975;58:183–91.

102. Bates ER, Stomel RJ, Hochman JS, Ohman EM. The use of intraaortic balloon counterpulsation as an adjunct to reperfusion therapy in cardiogenic shock. Int J Cardiol. 1998;65 Suppl 1:S37–42.

103. Sanborn TA, Sleeper LA, Bates ER, et al. Impact of thrombolysis, intra-aortic balloon pump counterpulsation, and their combination in cardiogenic shock complicating acute myocardial infarction: a report from the SHOCK Trial Registry. SHould we emergently revascularize Occluded Coronaries for cardiogenic shocK? J Am Coll Cardiol. 2000;36:1123–9.

104. Becker RC. Hemodynamic, mechanical, and metabolic determinants of thrombolytic efficacy: a theoretic framework for assessing the limitations of thrombolysis in patients with cardiogenic shock. Am Heart J. 1993;125:919–29.

105. Garber PJ, Mathieson AL, Ducas J, Patton JN, Geddes JS, Prewitt RM. Thrombolytic therapy in cardiogenic shock: effect of increased aortic pressure and rapid tPA administration. Can J Cardiol. 1995;11:30–6.

106. Hochman JS, Sleeper LA, Webb JG, et al. Early revascularization and long-term survival in cardiogenic shock complicating acute myocardial infarction. JAMA. 2006;295:2511–5.

107. Hochman JS, Sleeper LA, Webb JG, et al. Early revascularization in acute myocardial infarction complicated by cardiogenic shock. N Engl J Med. 1999;341:625–34.

108. Urban P, Stauffer JC, Bleed D, et al. A randomized evaluation of early revascularization to treat shock complicating acute myocardial infarction. The (Swiss) Multicenter Trial of Angioplasty for Shock-(S)MASH. Eur Heart J. 1999;20:1030–8.

# Chapter 3
# Arrhythmias

## Introduction

The physiologic impact of an arrhythmia depends on ventricular response rate, duration of arrhythmia, and underlying cardiac function. Bradyarrhythmias may decrease cardiac output due to heart rate alone in patients with a relatively fixed stroke volume. Loss of atrial contraction may cause a dramatic increase in pulmonary artery pressures in patients with hypertension and diastolic dysfunction. Similarly, tachyarrhythmias can decrease diastolic filling time and reduce cardiac output, resulting in hypotension and possible myocardial ischemia. The impact of a given arrhythmia depends on the patient's cardiac physiology and function. Treatment is determined by the hemodynamic insult. In this chapter, a systematic approach to diagnosis and evaluation of predisposing factors will be presented, followed by consideration of specific arrhythmias.

## Arrhythmia Diagnosis

### Basic Principles

The first principle in managing arrhythmias is to appropriately treat the patient, not the electrocardiogram. Accordingly, one must first decide whether the observed arrhythmia may be an artifact. If the arrhythmia is real and sustained, it must be determined whether it has important clinical consequences.

The next step is to establish the urgency of treatment. Clinical assessment includes evaluation of pulse, blood pressure, peripheral perfusion, and consideration of myocardial ischemia and/or congestive heart failure. If the patient loses consciousness or becomes hemodynamically unstable in the presence of a tachyarrhythmia other than sinus tachycardia, prompt cardioversion may be indicated

S. Hollenberg and S. Heitner, *Cardiology in Family Practice: A Practical Guide*,
Current Clinical Practice 1, DOI 10.1007/978-1-61779-385-1_3,
© Springer Science+Business Media, LLC 2012

regardless of anticoagulation status. If the patient is stable, there is often time to establish the rhythm diagnosis and decide upon the most appropriate treatment. Bradyarrhythmias produce less of a diagnostic challenge and treatment options are relatively straightforward.

The goals of antiarrhythmic therapy depend on the type of rhythm disturbance. The initial goal for the treatment of an arrhythmia is to stabilize the hemodynamics and ventricular response. The next goal is to restore sinus rhythm if possible. If restoration of sinus rhythm cannot be achieved, prevention of complications is important.

## Classification of Arrhythmias

Arrhythmias are usually classified according to anatomic origin, either supraventricular or ventricular. The most common supraventricular arrhythmia is sinus tachycardia, followed by atrial fibrillation, ectopic atrial or junctional tachycardia, multifocal atrial tachycardia, AV nodal reentry tachycardias, and accessory pathway tachycardias. Ventricular arrhythmias are most commonly premature ventricular beats, ventricular tachycardia and ventricular fibrillation.

It is sometimes useful to consider tachyarrhythmias from a treatment standpoint. Tachyarrhythmias that traverse the AV node can often be controlled by pharmacologically altering AV nodal conduction. Rhythms that traverse the AV node include atrial fibrillation and flutter, ectopic atrial and junctional tachycardias, multifocal atrial tachycardia, and AV nodal reentry tachycardias. Rhythms that do not utilize the AV node include accessory pathway tachycardias through a bypass tract, ventricular tachycardia, and ventricular fibrillation. When the arrhythmia does not utilize the AV node, slowing AV nodal conduction can be dangerous.

## Rhythm Diagnosis

A comprehensive description of the diagnosis of arrhythmias is beyond the scope of this manuscript. A 12-lead electrocardiogram with a long rhythm strip and a previously obtained 12-lead electrocardiogram for comparison are ideal; if a previous EKG is not available, a systematic approach using a current 12-lead EKG is essential. An approach is outlined using the following five steps [1].

1. Locate the p-wave.
   p-Waves are often best seen in leads II and $V_1$. Normal p-waves are upright in leads II, III and aVF, and may be biphasic in leads II and $V_1$. If p-waves are present and always followed by a QRS complex, the rhythm is most likely sinus tachycardia, which usually occurs at a rate between 100 and 180 in adults. Ectopic atrial and junctional tachycardias often present with negative p-waves in leads II, III and

aVF. If p-waves are present and the rhythm is irregular, the rhythm is most likely atrial fibrillation. If the p-wave is buried in the QRS or ST segment, the rhythm is most likely AV nodal reentry tachycardia, which usually present with atrial rates from 140 to 220. If there are multiple p-waves followed by a single QRS, especially if the atrial rate is near 300, the rhythm is most likely atrial flutter. If no p-waves are present, the rhythm is most likely atrial fibrillation.

2. Establish the relationship between the p-wave and QRS.

If there are more p-waves than QRS complexes, then AV block is present. If there are more QRS complexes than p-waves, the rhythm is likely an accelerated junctional or ventricular rhythm. If the relationship of the p-wave and QRS is 1:1, then measurement of the PR interval can yield useful diagnostic clues.

3. Examine the QRS morphology.

A narrow QRS complex (<0.12 ms) indicates a supraventricular arrhythmia. A wide QRS complex can be either ventricular tachycardia or supraventricular tachycardia with either a pre-existing bundle branch block, or, less commonly, aberrant ventricular conduction or an antegrade accessory pathway.

4. Search for other clues.

The clues to guide appropriate therapy depend on the situation. Carotid sinus massage increases AV block and can either break a supraventricular tachycardia or bring out previously undetected flutter waves. Any patient with a ventricular rate of exactly 150 beats/min should be suspected of having atrial flutter with 2–1 AV block. A rate greater than 200 beats/min in an otherwise healthy adult should raise the suspicion of an accessory pathway. Severe left axis deviation (−60 to 120°) during tachycardia suggests a ventricular origin, as does AV dissociation, fusion beats (which result from simultaneous activation of two foci, one ventricular and one supraventricular), and capture beats (beats that capture the ventricles and are conducted with a narrow complex, ruling out fixed bundle branch block). Grouped beating or more p-waves than QRS complexes suggests the possibility of second-degree AV block.

5. Establish the rhythm in the clinical setting.

# Atrial Fibrillation

## *Etiology and Pathophysiology*

Atrial fibrillation is the most common sustained tachycardia encountered in clinical practice. It is estimated that 2.2 million Americans have paroxysmal or persistent atrial fibrillation. The prevalence increases with age and is more common in men than in women [2]. The prevalence is 3.8% for persons over 60 years old and 9.0% for persons over 80 years old [2].

Atrial fibrillation is characterized by uncoordinated atrial activity with an irregular ventricular response, usually rapid (see Fig. 3.1). Atrial fibrillation can occur with or without underlying structural heart disease or may be secondary to other

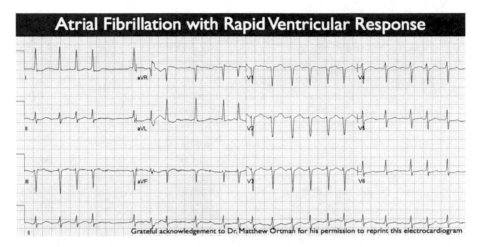

**Fig. 3.1** Atrial fibrillation. ECG courtesy of Matthew Ortman, MD

predisposing conditions. Cardiac diseases associated with atrial fibrillation include hypertension, valvular heart disease, coronary artery disease, and cardiomyopathies. Atrial fibrillation has also been linked to alcohol ingestion, pulmonary embolism, hyperthyroidism, obstructive sleep apnea, chronic obstructive pulmonary disease, and is common following cardiac or thoracic surgery. Atrial fibrillation following an acute MI carries a poor prognostic sign [3].

Atrial fibrillation has been classified as paroxysmal, persistent, permanent, and lone [4]. Two or more episodes of atrial fibrillation has been defined as recurrent atrial fibrillation. Recurrent atrial fibrillation is further classified as either paroxysmal (terminates spontaneously) or persistent (sustained and does not convert to sinus rhythm without either pharmacological or electrical cardioversion). Permanent atrial fibrillation refers to long-standing atrial fibrillation (greater than 1 year) in which cardioversion has not been indicated or attempted [4]. Lone atrial fibrillation refers to patients without structural heart disease or conditions predisposing to atrial fibrillation.

The mechanism of atrial fibrillation is not entirely clear. The conventional viewpoint was that multiple reentrant impulses wandering throughout the atria creates continuous electrical activity, the multiple wavelet hypothesis [5]. More recently, focal origin from electrically active tissue situated in the pulmonary veins has been identified [6]. Other foci include the right atrium, superior vena cava, and coronary sinus [6–8]. The distinction between these mechanisms is more than merely academic, since origin from discrete foci presents the possibility of treatment either by ablating these foci or isolating them from the rest of the atrium.

Atrial fibrillation results in loss of effective atrial contraction and atrioventricular (AV) synchrony. The variation in the RR interval leads to changing diastolic filling intervals, and therefore, varying stroke volumes of AV synchrony may have an adverse impact on cardiac output.

## Clinical Features

The symptoms of atrial fibrillation result from the rapidity and irregularity of the ventricular response and the loss of AV synchrony. The most common symptoms include palpitations, dyspnea, fatigue, lightheadedness, chest pain, and syncope. However, some patients with atrial fibrillation are completely asymptomatic.

The initial workup should include a complete history and physical exam, ECG, thyroid function tests, chest radiograph, complete blood count, serum electrolytes, and transthoracic echocardiogram. The history should focus on the onset, duration, frequency, symptoms, precipitating or reversible factors, and terminating events of each episode.

The ECG shows absent p-wave and an irregularly irregular rhythm. Fibrillatory waves may be seen in the inferior leads, at a rate of 300–700 beats/min. The ventricular rate is usually between 100 and 180 beats/min, but may be slower if there is AV nodal conduction disease, high vagal tone, or drugs affecting AV nodal conduction. The ventricular rate may be regular if the patient is ventricular paced or there is an AV block. A chest X-ray is useful to evaluate the lungs, cardiac silhouette, and pulmonary vasculature.

All patients with new onset atrial fibrillation should be evaluated by echocardiography. Echocardiography should be performed to evaluate the left and right atrial size, left and right ventricular size and function, valvular abnormalities or pericardial disease. Transthoracic echocardiography can occasionally detect left atrial thrombus but the sensitivity is low. Transesophageal echocardiography is the most sensitive and specific technique for diagnosing a thrombus in the left atrium, and should be considered before cardioversion or after a suspected embolic event.

Exercise testing should be performed on patients with suspected ischemic heart disease and those being considered for type IC antiarrhythmic drug therapy [4]. Holter or event monitors may be used to capture the arrhythmia in patients with paroxysmal atrial fibrillation and to evaluate rate control.

## Therapy

The three goals of therapy for atrial fibrillation are to control the rate, to restore and maintain normal sinus rhythm, and to prevent complications. Recent clinical trials have created controversy concerning whether rhythm control is superior to rate control. The Atrial Fibrillation Follow-up Investigation of Rhythm Management (AFFIRM) study enrolled 4,060 patients older than 65 with at least one risk factor for stroke or death in a randomized controlled trial comparing a rhythm control strategy to rate control [9]. Patients were randomized to antiarrhythmic drugs or cardioversion to restore sinus rhythm, or AV nodal blocking agents. The rate control groups were anticoagulated indefinitely. The rhythm control groups were anticoagulated, but at the discretion of their physician could be stopped if they were in normal sinus rhythm for longer than 4 weeks. The composite endpoint (death, disabling stroke, disabling anoxic encephalopathy, major bleeding, cardiac arrest) were not statistically different, but overall mortality was higher in the rhythm control group, although this was not statistically significant. The rhythm control group had more hospitalization, and in a 5-year follow-up, only 63% were in normal sinus rhythm. Stroke rates averaged 1% per year in both groups, and occurred mostly in patients who stopped taking warfarin or who were subtherapeutic [9].

The Rate Control vs. Electrical Cardioversion for Persistent Atrial Fibrillation (RACE) study was a similar randomized control trial comparing rhythm vs. rate control in 522 patients with persistent atrial fibrillation, 90% of whom had risk factors for stroke [10]. Patients in the rate control group received beta blockers, calcium channel blockers, or digoxin, and those in the rhythm group were cardioverted and maintained on sotalol. All patients received anticoagulation, but this could be discontinued in the rhythm control group if sinus rhythm was achieved. There was no statistically significant difference in the composite endpoint (cardiovascular mortality, heart failure, thromboembolic events, bleeding, pacemaker implantation, drug side effects) in the rate control (17.2%) and rhythm control (22.6%) groups [10]. As with the AFFIRM trial, there were increased thromboembolic complications in the rhythm group, mainly among patients who discontinued anticoagulation therapy.

The Pharmacological Intervention in Atrial Fibrillation (PIAF) study was a rate vs. rhythm trial enrolling 252 patients with persistent symptomatic atrial fibrillation, with symptomatic improvement as the primary end point [11]. The rate control group was given diltiazem, while the rhythm group was given amiodarone; all patients were anticoagulated. Quality of life and symptoms improved in both groups to the same extent. The rhythm group had better exercise tolerance. More patients in the rhythm control group were hospitalized and they suffered more drug side effects.

The Strategies of Treatment of Atrial Fibrillation (STAF) pilot study examined the effects of rate vs. rhythm control on death, cardiovascular events, cardiopulmonary resuscitation or systemic emboli [12]. The rate control group received an AV nodal blocking medication (beta blocker, calcium channel blocker, digoxin). The rhythm control group received amiodarone or some other Class I antiarrhythmic, or electrical cardioversion. Both groups were anticoagulated. There was no statistically significant difference in either the primary endpoint or the secondary endpoints (syncope, bleeding, worsening heart failure, quality of life). The rhythm control group required more frequent hospitalizations with longer lengths of stay. At a 3-year follow-up, only 23% of the rhythm control group were in sinus rhythm [12].

Based on these trials, either a rate control or a rhythm control strategy can be chosen, individualized to a particular patient. The initial priority in a patient presenting with atrial fibrillation is to control the ventricular rate acutely. This can be accomplished with either beta blockers or calcium channel blockers. If very rapid control is required, intravenous beta blockade with metoprolol (5 mg IV every 5 min up to 3 doses) or esmolol (500 mcg/kg bolus and 50 mcg/kg/min infusion titrated up in 50 mcg/kg/min increments every 3–5 min up to 200 mcg/kg/min), followed by oral therapy can be used. Risks include hypotension, bronchospasm, and negative inotropic effects. Intravenous calcium channel blockade with diltiazem (10–20 mg IV over 2 min and then at 5–20 mg/h IV) or verapamil (2.5 mg IV over 2 min, repeated every 15 min up to 15 mg), followed by oral therapy is equally acceptable. Risks include hypotension and heart failure. Digoxin is a second line alternative that is much better for chronic than acute rate control, and is recommended in patients with heart failure [13]. Digoxin can be loaded intravenously (1 mg load, usually 0.25 mg IV every 6 h but can be given as 0.5 mg once followed by 0.25 mg every 3 h for 2 doses) if necessary. Measurement of levels should be done at steady state, and is not especially helpful in atrial fibrillation except in patients with suspected toxicity. Maintenance doses range from 0.125 to 0.375 mg/day, and require adjustment for renal insufficiency.

Chronically, rate control is needed to avoid the symptoms and hemodynamic instability caused by a rapid ventricular response. Beta blockers (atenolol, metoprolol, propranolol, esmolol), nondihydropyridine calcium antagonists (verapamil, diltiazem), and digoxin slow AV nodal conduction and are the recommended pharmacologic agents for rate control. The current ACC/AHA/ESC guidelines recommend dose titration to a resting heart rate of 60–80 and 90–115 beats/min during exercise [4]. Digoxin provides rate control at rest but not with exercise, and is used in combination with beta blockers or calcium blockers or alone when they are not tolerated.

Hemodynamically unstable patients require emergent cardioversion, and those with acute heart failure or angina should be considered for urgent cardioversion. Electrical cardioversion may be more effective when the defibrillator pads are placed in an anterior/posterior orientation to direct the current through the atria.

Rhythm control is achieved either through synchronized external cardioversion or pharmacological cardioversion. The risk of thromboembolism is the same for electrical and pharmacological cardioversion. If the duration of atrial fibrillation is less than 48 h then the patient is at low thromboembolic risk; the patient should be heparinized, cardioverted and given aspirin for 1 month. A patient at high risk (mitral valve disease, previous thromboembolism, severe LV dysfunction) should be anticoagulated for 1 month before elective cardioversion. For patients having atrial fibrillation for more than 48 h or of unknown duration, intravenous heparin and oral warfarin should be initiated upon presentation. Transesophageal echocardiography can be used to evaluate for left atrial thrombus. If no thrombus is visualized, the patient can be safely cardioverted and then anticoagulated for 1 month [14], since recovery of atrial mechanical function may be delayed despite restoration of sinus rhythm. If a thrombus is seen, the patient should be anticoagulated for at least 3–4 weeks prior to elective cardioversion.

The use of pharmacologic cardioversion should be based upon the duration of the atrial fibrillation, presence or absence of structural heart disease, and persistent symptoms on rate control agents. Before instituting an antiarrhythmic agent, reversible causes (hyperthyroidism, hypertension, heart failure, cardiac surgery, pulmonary embolism) need to be addressed.

Antiarrhythmic agents are divided into classes according to mechanism of action. Class I agents are sodium channel blockers and prolong the QT interval, leading to the potential for proarrhythmia and torsades de pointes. Class IA agents, which include quinidine, procainamide, and disopyramide, block potassium channels as well. Quinidine can cause sinus and AV nodal blockade, in addition to its proarrhythmic effects. When initiating this agent, the patient should have continuous electocardiographic monitoring. Noncardiac effects include abdominal cramping, nausea, and diarrhea, and cinchonism, a constellation of symptoms (tinnitus, hearing loss, blurred vision, delirium, confusion, and psychosis) associated with high plasma levels of the drug. Procainamide side effects include lupus-like syndrome, nausea, vomiting dizziness, psychosis, headache, depression, vasculitis, myalgias, fever, and pancytopenia or agranulocytosis, which may be life-threatening. Procainamide can also lengthen the PR interval in patients with AV conduction disease. The drug has an active metabolite (N-acetylprocainamide, or NAPA), and should be adjusted in renal or hepatic impairment. Disopyramide has negative inotropic effects and should be avoided in patients with heart failure, and is anticholinergic symptoms and should not be used in patients with glaucoma, myasthenia gravis, or urinary retention. Disopyramide needs to be adjusted for renal and hepatic impairment.

Class IC antiarrhythmic agents (flecainide, propafenone, moricizine) block sodium channels but have less profound effects on repolarization. All Class IC agents have a negative inotropic effect and therefore are contraindicated in patients with heart failure. Extracardiac effects of flecainide include dizziness, headache, blurred vision, and ataxia. Propafenone has beta blocking effects in addition to Class IC antiarrhythmic properties, and should be avoided in patients with reactive airway diseases and sinus node dysfunction. Other common side effects include nausea, metallic taste, increased liver enzymes, dizziness, and constipation.

Class III antiarrhythmic agents (amiodarone, sotalol, dofetilide, ibutilide) are potassium channel blockers and prolong repolarization, action potential durations and refractory periods. All Class III agents increase the QT interval and may precipitate torsades de pointes. Amiodarone blocks potassium, sodium, and calcium channels, and alpha and beta receptors. Amiodarone is highly lipid soluble and accumulates in high concentrations in adipose tissue and highly perfused organs, such as the lung, liver, and skin. Because of the extensive accumulation, the elimination half-life is long after discontinuation of the drug. The adverse effects of amiodarone therapy include pulmonary fibrosis, thyroid dysfunction, AV node blockade, hepatotoxicity, corneal microdeposits, optic nerve injury, gray–blue skin discoloration, tremor, ataxia, and peripheral neuropathy. Amiodarone interacts with other drugs, notably warfarin and digoxin, mandating dose adjustments if taken together. Liver function tests, thyroid function tests, and pulmonary function should be monitored periodically in patients on amiodarone [15]. Sotalol is a racemic mixture of d and l isomers that has Class III and beta blocker actions. Side effects are largely due to the beta blockade, mandating caution in patients with reactive airway disease, sinus bradycardia, AV block, and uncontrolled heart failure. Sotalol has proarrhythmic affects and should not be administered to patients with prolonged QT intervals; initiation of sotalol is performed in a hospital setting with continuous cardiac monitoring. Sotalol is excreted by the kidneys and the dose should be adjusted in renal impairment. Dofetilide blocks the rapid component of the delayed rectifier potassium current, and prolongs the repolarization and refractory period in the atrium and ventricles without affecting the conduction system. Dofetilide prolongs the QT interval, and poses a risk of developing torsades de pointes, which is greatest within the first 3 days of drug initiation, so the drug is started in the hospital with continuous cardiac monitoring. Dofetilide is renally eliminated and interacts with a number of drugs, including verapamil, cimetidine, diuretics, keto-conazole, macrolide antibiotics, trimethoprim, triamterene, metformin, amiloride, and megestrol. Ibutilide is an intravenous Class III antiarrhythmic drug which is used to terminate acute atrial fibrillation acutely. One milligram of ibutilide should be infused over 10 min. Termination of the arrhythmia should occur within 60 min of initiating the dose, and if the arrhythmia does not terminate, the dose may be repeated. Like all class III agents, ibutilide can lengthen the QT interval and precipi-tate torsades de pointes, and so continuous electrocardiographic monitoring for 6 h after drug administration is mandatory, even if sinus rhythm has been restored.

The choice of an antiarrhythmic agent depends on the clinical setting. Propafenone or flecainide are recommended as first-line drugs for pharmacologic cardioversion in patients without structural heart disease, although amiodarone, sotalol, and dofetilide are alternative agents [4]. Sotalol and amiodarone can be used for adren-ergically mediated atrial fibrillation, and disopyramide is suggested for vagally-induced atrial fibrillation. In patients with structural heart disease, amiodarone and sotalol are recommended as the first-line drugs. Class IC antiarrhythmic agents (flecainide, encainide, moricizine) should be avoided in patients with coronary heart disease due to the increased mortality shown in the CAST trial [4, 5, 16, 17]. Amiodarone is recommended for patients with heart failure and atrial fibrillation; dofetilide is an alternative [4].

The other important issue in the management of patients with atrial fibrillation is prevention of complications, most notably stroke. Atrial fibrillation is a risk factor for stroke, but varies among patients. The annual risk in the Framingham study was 4.2% but may be higher for patients with more than one risk factor [18]. Two studies, Atrial Fibrillation Investigation (AFI) [19] and Stroke Prevention in Atrial Fibrillation (SPAF) [20] identified individual risk factors that increased the risk of stroke in patients with atrial fibrillation. Risk factors for stroke in the AFI study included previous stroke, hypertension, diabetes, and advanced age. SPAF corre-lated stroke risk with previous stroke, females over the age 75, systolic hyperten-sion, and low ejection fraction. To simplify the system, Gage et al. combined the risk factors from both studies devised a point system called CHADS2 [21]. Two points were given to a history of previous stroke, and CHF, hypertension, age >75, and diabetes were given one point. A score of 0–1 was identified as low risk for stroke and warfarin was not recommended. A score of 2–3 was moderate risk and 4–6 was high risk. Warfarin was recommended for both the moderate and high risk groups (see Fig. 3.1).

A new and recently FDA-approved alternative to warfarin for thomboprophy-laxis in patients with atrial fibrillation is the direct thrombin inhibitor dabigatran. In the RE-LY study, dabigatran given at a dose of 110 mg was associated with rates of stroke and systemic embolism that were similar to those seen in the warfarin arm, but with lower rates of major hemorrhage. Dabigatran administered at a dose of 150 mg (the current dose approved by the FDA for thromboprophylaxis in atrial fibrillation) [22], as compared with warfarin, was associated with lower rates of stroke and systemic embolism but similar rates of major hemorrhage [23] (Fig. 3.2).

# The CHADS$_2$ Index
## Stroke Risk Score for Atrial Fibrillation

| | Score (points) | Risk of Stroke (%/year) | |
|---|---|---|---|
| | 0 | 1.9 | |
| | 1 | 2.8 | |
| Approximate Risk threshold for Anticoagulation | | ......................................... | 3%/year |
| | 2 | 4.0 | |
| | 3 | 5.9 | |
| | 4 | 8.5 | |
| | 5 | 12.5 | |
| | 6 | 18.2 | |

**Fig. 3.2**  Stroke risk in patients with atrial fibrillation

The ACC/AHA/ESC developed their own risk-based approach to antithrombotic therapy in patients with atrial fibrillation (Table 3.1). These guidelines recommend

**Table 3.1**  Risk-based approach to antithrombotic therapy in patients with atrial fibrillation (Adapted from Fuster et al. [4])

| Patient features | Antithrombotic therapy |
|---|---|
| Age <60, no heart disease | Aspirin 325 mg/day or no therapy |
| Age <60, heart disease but no risk factors [a] | Aspirin 325 mg/day |
| Age >60, no risk factors [a] | Aspirin 325 mg/day |
| Age >60 with diabetes or CAD | Warfarin (INR 2–3) |
| | Addition of aspirin, 81–162 mg/day is optional |
| Age >75, especially women | Warfarin (INR approximately 2) |
| Heart failure (EF <35%) | Warfarin (INR 2–3) |
| Thyrotoxicosis | |
| Hypertension | |
| Rheumatic heart disease | Warfarin (INR 2.5–3.5) |
| Prosthetic heart valves | |
| Prior thromboembolism | |
| Persistent atrial thrombus on TEE | |

*INR* international normalized ratio; *CAD* coronary artery disease; *EF* ejection fraction; *TEE* transesophageal echocardiography
[a] Risk factors for thromboembolism include heart failure, ejection fraction less than 35%, and a history of hypertension

warfarin for patients with atrial fibrillation and valvular disease, previous stroke, or at least one risk factor (heart failure, female over the age of 75, low ejection fraction, diabetes, hypertension). Aspirin is recommended for patients below 60 years of age with no risk factors with or without heart disease and patients above 60 years of age with no heart disease and no risk factors. The target INR range for nonvalvular atrial fibrillation is 2–3, and 2.5–3.5 for valvular disease [4].

Whether anticoagulation can be stopped in patients who have converted to sinus rhythm is a difficult and unresolved question. The results of the rate control vs. rhythm control strategies described above suggest that patients who have been converted to sinus rhythm may have paroxysmal episodes of atrial fibrillation that go undetected. On the other hand, anticoagulation poses a risk of hemorrhage. In general, chronic anticoagulation with warfarin is desirable unless the patient is at low risk for stroke or the drug is contraindicated [13].

Nonpharmacological therapies (surgical ablation, percutaneous catheter ablation) are indicated for patients who are symptomatic and refractory to medical therapy. Foci in the pulmonary veins, superior vena cava, right and left atrium or coronary sinus can be ablated percutaneously using a radiofrequency catheter. The risk of recurrence after focal ablation is currently about 30–50%, and many patients still require antiarrhythmic therapy after ablation [4]. Complications of catheter ablation include pulmonary vein stenosis, pericardial effusion and tamponade, phrenic nerve paralysis, and systemic embolism. Catheter ablation of the AV node with insertion of a permanent pacemaker is another option. A meta-analysis concluded that AV nodal ablation and pacemaker implantation improved symptoms, quality of life, exercise duration, and left ventricular function [24]. Surgical ablation, the Maze procedure, is an invasive approach that requires a thoracotomy and general anesthesia. This option is usually employed in patients requiring open-heart surgery for other indications.

# Supraventricular Tachycardia

## *Sinus Tachycardia*

Sinus tachycardia is a rhythm which arises from the SA node with a heart rate >100 beats/min. It is usually a physiologic response to an underlying cause, which can include pain, anxiety, fever, exercise, hyperthyroidism, volume depletion, hypotension, pulmonary embolism, myocardial infarction, anemia, or infection. Certain illicit drugs, such as cocaine, amphetamines, and ecstasy can precipitate this arrhythmia. Other stimulants (caffeine, alcohol, nicotine) and prescribed medications (atropine, catecholamines, aminophylline, doxorubicin, daunorubicin) can induce sinus tachycardia.

Occasional patients may have inappropriate sinus tachycardia, an uncommon arrhythmia that occurs most commonly in young women, and a disproportionate number from the health care profession. The mechanism is unclear; studies have suggested that there is abnormal sinus node automaticity or excess sympathetic and reduced parasympathetic tone [25, 26]. Diagnostic criteria include exclusion of secondary causes.

Patients may be asymptomatic or may complain of palpitations, lightheadedness, or dizziness. The p-waves have the same sinus morphology (upright in leads I–III). With increasing heart rate, the PR interval decreases. The QRS complex is narrow. Vagal maneuvers (carotid massage or Valsalva maneuver) may help in differentiating sinus tachycardia from other paroxysmal supraventricular tachycardias.

The first priority in the treatment of sinus tachycardia is to identify the underlying cause. Once the cause is identified, treatment can be tailored to that cause. Pharmacologic therapy can be used in certain situations. Beta blockers may be used to treat sinus tachycardia due to anxiety, hyperthyroidism, and myocardial infarction. For inappropriate sinus tachycardia beta blockers are first-line therapy, with calcium blockers as an alternative [26]. Calcium blockers can be substituted if beta blockers are contraindicated. If patients are refractory to medical therapy, sinus node modification by catheter ablation is an option.

## Focal (Ectopic) Atrial Tachycardia

Repetitive focal atrial tachycardia is thought to be caused by enhanced automaticity arising from a single atrial focus. This arrhythmia is seen in patients with organic heart disease, lung disease, myocardial infarction, infection, electrolyte disturbances (hypokalemia), and hypoxemia. Medications that can enhance automaticity include digoxin and theophylline. Drugs of abuse such as cocaine, and alcohol can also induce this arrhythmia.

On the ECG, the p-wave morphology will be consistent but different from the sinus p-waves. The QRS complex is usually narrow. There is often a progressive acceleration in the atrial rate (warm up) at the beginning followed by a gradual decrease at the end of the arrhythmia (cool down).

For acute treatment in hemodynamically stable patients, either adenosine, beta blockers, or conversion with intravenous antiarrhythmics from Classes IA, IC, or III is recommended [26]. Hemodynamically unstable patients should be cardioverted. If rate regulation only is needed in the acute setting, intravenous beta blockers, verapamil, or diltiazem is indicated. Digoxin can also be used as long as the arrhythmia is not due to digoxin toxicity. For prophylactic therapy to prevent recurrence, beta blockers and calcium channel blockers are the treatment of choice. Disopyramide, flecainide, propafenone, sotalol, and amiodarone are alternatives for prophylactic treatment [26]. Class IC antiarrhythmic should not be given to patients with coronary artery disease. For symptomatic patients refractory to medical therapy, catheter ablation is recommended.

## Multifocal Atrial Tachycardia

Multifocal atrial tachycardia (MAT) usually occurs in the acutely ill, elderly patient, or in those with pulmonary disease [27]. MAT is also associated with diabetes, hypokalemia, hypomagnesemia, chronic kidney disease, hypoxia, acidosis, hypercapnia, and certain medications. MAT is diagnosed by the presence of three or more different p-wave morphologies on one EKG with an irregularly irregular rhythm. The most useful therapy for MAT is to treat the underlying causes, including hypoxemia and hypercapnia, myocardial ischemia, congestive heart failure, or electrolyte disturbances. Beta blockers and calcium channels blockers can slow an excessive ventricular rate [28]. These agents should be used cautiously in patients with known congestive heart failure or reduced left ventricular function.

## AV Nodal Reentry Tachycardia

Atrioventricular nodal reentry tachycardia (AVNRT) is the most common paroxysmal supraventricular tachycardia, accounting for about 60% of all supraventricular arrhythmias [29]. It tends to be more common in women than men. Symptoms emerge most commonly in young adults, although they can occur at any age. Most patients with AVNRT do not have structural heart disease.

Dual AV nodal pathways with different conduction velocities and refractory periods are usually present, setting up the substrate for reentry [30]. The slow pathway has a short refractory time, and the fast pathway has a longer refractory time. A normal sinus beat travels down both fast and slow pathways. In the most common variant, slow–fast AVNRT, a critically timed premature beat finds that the fast pathway is still refractory, and conducts down the slow pathway. If the fast pathway has recovered, the impulse can then be conducted retrograde up the fast pathway to the atrium, creating a reentrant circuit. The uncommon fast-slow AVNRT has antegrade conduction down the fast pathway and retrograde conduction up the slow pathway.

The symptoms of AVNRT are related to the rapid heart rate and include palpitations, lightheadedness, dizziness, and sometimes syncope. Some patients may experience chest pain or dyspnea. The heart rate ranges from 120 to 220 beats/min. The p-wave can occur immediately before or after the QRS complex, or may not be seen on the electrocardiogram due to near-simultaneous retrograde atrial and antegrade ventricular activation. If p-wave occurs immediately after the QRS, there may be a pseudo-R wave in $V_1$ or pseudo-S wave leads II, III, and aVF reflecting retrograde conduction. In the less common fast-slow AVNRT, the p-wave may occur just before the next QRS.

Carotid sinus massage or other vagal maneuvers may convert AVNRT to normal sinus rhythm. Adenosine 6–12 mg IV is the preferred initial drug treatment because its extremely short half-life minimizes side effects. The 12 mg dose may be repeated if necessary. Urgent cardioversion may be necessary with circulatory insufficiency. The AV node action potential is calcium channel dependent, which make verapamil or diltiazem very effective in terminating this arrhythmia. Beta blockers are also effective.

For chronic therapy in patients with frequent symptomatic episodes, beta blockers are preferred since they suppress the initiating premature atrial contractions. Calcium channel blockers and digoxin can also be used. In patients who do not respond to AV nodal blocking agents and do not have structural heart disease, flecainide or propafenone are the recommended antiarrhythmic drugs of choice [26].

Radiofrequency catheter ablation of the slow pathway is a curative treatment modality in patients with AVNRT. In the North American Society for Pacing and Electrophysiology (NASPE) prospective registry, the success rate was 96.1%, with AV block as a complication in only 1% [31]. Based on these results, and with appropriate selection by physicians, many patients with recurrent AVNRT are choosing catheter ablation therapy over antiarrhythmic therapy.

## Atrioventricular Reciprocating Tachycardia

Atrioventricular reciprocating tachycardia (AVRT) is characterized by an extranodal accessory bypass tract connecting the atrium to the ventricles. Approximately 30% of patients with supraventricular tachycardia will be found to have an accessory pathway [29].

Conduction through these accessory pathways can be from the atrium to the ventricles (antegrade conduction) or from the ventricles to the atrium (retrograde conduction). When conduction goes down the AV node and back up the bypass tract, the QRS complex is narrow and conduction is termed orthodromic [29]. When conduction goes down the bypass tract and back up the AV node, the QRS complex is wide and conduction is termed antidromic [29].

Accessory pathways that are capable of antegrade conduction pre-excite the ventricles. The characteristic ECG finding of this pre-excitation is the delta wave. Patients with a delta wave and an atrioventricular reentry tachycardia are said to have Wolff–Parkinson–White (WPW) syndrome. There are no characteristic ECG findings when the accessory pathway conducts in the retrograde direction. These pathways are termed concealed accessory pathways.

In AVRT, a critically timed premature atrial or ventricular beat initiates a reentrant tachycardia. Orthodromic AVRT uses the AV node and His–Purkinje system to conduct the impulse to the ventricles; the QRS complex is narrow, and the heart rate ranges from 150 to 250 beats/min. In antidromic AVRT, the impulses are conducted to the ventricle through the accessory pathway, generating a wide QRS complex. Antidromic AVRT is faster, because of the relatively short refractory period of the accessory pathway.

### Wolff–Parkinson–White Syndrome

WPW syndrome is a pre-excitation syndrome characterized by an accessory pathway (bundle of Kent) that bypasses the AV node and activates the ventricles prematurely. Most patients with WPW have otherwise normal hearts, but some have

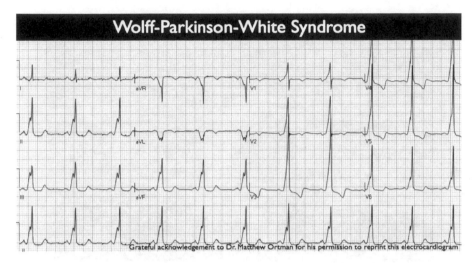

**Fig. 3.3** Wolfe–Parkinson–White syndrome, with a delta wave indicative of fusion between conduction down the His pathway and conduction down the accessory pathway. ECG courtesy of Matthew Ortman, MD

congenital anomalies, such as Ebstein's anomaly, septal defects, transposition of the great vessels, and a familial form of hypertrophic cardiomyopathy. The prevalence of WPW syndrome is approximately 0.1–0.3% of the general population. WPW is twice as common in men as in women.

The electrocardiographic findings include a shortened PR interval, delta wave and a widened QRS complex (see Fig. 3.3). The PR interval is short due to the rapid AV conduction through the accessory pathway, bypassing the delay in the AV node. The delta wave is produced by the slow early activation of the ventricles by the accessory pathway. The widened QRS complex results from fusion of early ventricular activation by the accessory pathway and activation from the impulses conducted through the AV node and infranodal system (see Fig. 3.4).

Most patients with WPW syndrome present with symptoms of tachyarrhythmias. Tachyarrhythmias associated with WPW syndrome include AVRT, atrial fibrillation, atrial flutter, and ventricular fibrillation. Approximately 10–30% of patients with WPW will develop atrial fibrillation [32]. In those patients, AVRT usually precedes atrial fibrillation. The impulses generated during atrial fibrillation can conduct antegrade down the accessory pathway, and can be transmitted at very high rates (>250 beats/min) due to the short refractory time of the accessory pathway.

The ECG in atrial fibrillation with WPW is characteristic (see Fig. 3.5). The diagnosis is made by the irregularly irregular rhythm, which indicates atrial fibrillation, and the varying width of the QRS complexes – which is caused by varying degrees of fusion resulting from antegrade conduction down both the normal conducting system and the bypass tract. Some of the R–R intervals can be extremely short, less than 250 ms. Rapid atrial fibrillation in WPW is very dangerous because it can deteriorate to ventricular fibrillation and sudden cardiac death.

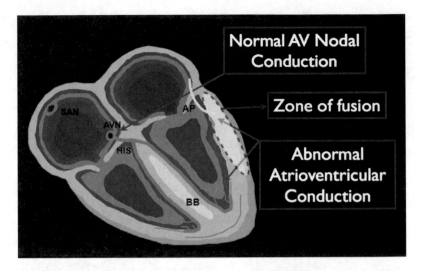

**Fig. 3.4** Mechanism of fusion in Wolfe–Parkinson–White syndrome. The QRS complex varies in width depending on the balance between conduction down the AV node and conduction down the accessory pathway. *SAN* sinoatrial node; *AVN* atrioventricular node; *HIS* bundle of His; *BB* bundle branches; *AP* accessory pathway

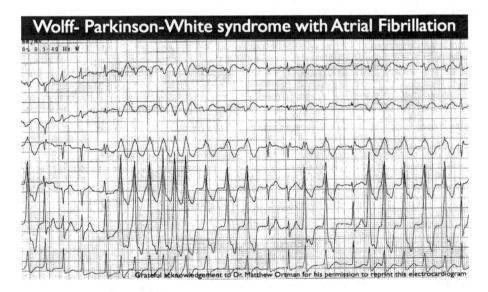

**Fig. 3.5** Atrial fibrillation in the setting of Wolfe–Parkinson–White syndrome. The rhythm is irregular, and differential fusion causes the QRS width to vary among beats. ECG courtesy of Matthew Ortman, MD

**Therapy**

Pharmacologic treatment of AVRT must be tailored to the electrophysiologic properties of the arrhythmia. Therapy of orthodromic accessory pathway reentrant tachycardias entails AV nodal blockade with vagal maneuvers, IV adenosine, and calcium channel blockers [26]. Second line drugs include intravenous procainamide and beta blockers. Chronic therapy for orthodromic AVRT usually involves administration of Class IC antiarrhythmic drugs (flecainide, encainide).

For antidromic accessory pathway reentrant tachycardias, intravenous procainamide is the drug of choice because it slows conduction down the accessory pathway. Atrial flutter or fibrillation with antidromic conduction is a dangerous situation due to the potential for extremely rapid conduction down the accessory pathway with resultant rapid ventricular rates. In this situation, the ventricular rate is modulated by competition between AV nodal conduction and conduction down the bypass tract. Drugs that block the AV node such as digoxin, verapamil, or diltiazem can thus increase ventricular rate and lead to the potential for ventricular fibrillation. In both orthodromic and antidromic AVRT, cardioversion is indicated for hemodynamic collapse.

For chronic therapy of antidromic AVRT, Class IC antiarrhythmic drugs are recommended [26]. AAVRT Amiodarone and Class IA agents can be used as second line therapy.

Catheter ablation is potentially curative, and has a low complication rate [33, 34]. Catheter ablation was given a Class I recommendation by the ACC/AHA/ESC for patients with WPW syndrome and symptomatic arrhythmias, atrial fibrillation or poorly tolerated AVRT [26]. The same group gave catheter ablation a Class IIa recommendation for asymptomatic patients in high-risk occupations. Many patients with recurrent arrhythmias choose catheter ablation over life-long antiarrhythmic medication, although recurrences after ablation do occur [34].

## Junctional Tachycardia

Junctional tachycardias are rare and usually benign. They result from increased automaticity arising from a high junctional focus or triggered activity [35]. Nonparoxysmal junctional tachycardia is usually caused by digoxin toxicity, hypokalemia, theophylline, inferior wall myocardial infarctions, myocarditis, catecholamine excess, or post-cardiac surgery.

The ECG shows a narrow complex tachycardia with absent p-waves and a heart rate ranging from 70 to 110 beats/min. Onset is usually gradual with a typical "warm-up" and "cool-down" pattern. If digoxin toxicity is the etiology, the ECG may show a second degree Mobitz type I block.

Management for junctional tachycardia is to eliminate and correct the underlying cause. Occasionally, loss of AV synchrony leads to decreased cardiac output. Overdrive atrial pacing at an appropriate rate can improve AV synchrony and cardiac output. Persistent junctional tachycardia can be treated with beta blockers or calcium channel blockers [35].

## Ventricular Tachycardia

Ventricular tachyarrhythmias (VT) can be classified as benign or malignant. The chief distinction, in addition to duration and hemodynamic consequences, is the presence of significant structural heart disease. This distinction is especially important when evaluating premature ventricular contractions (PVCs) and nonsustained ventricular tachycardia (NSVT). In patients without structural heart disease, the risk of sudden death or hemodynamic compromise is minimal, and therapy is rarely necessary in the absence of symptoms. In patients with coronary artery disease, a history of myocardial infarction, or cardiomyopathy, PVCs may indicate the potential for malignant ventricular tachyarrhythmias and merit prompt and thorough assessment. Prompt evaluation for and reversal of precipitating factors such as ischemia and electrolyte abnormalities are indicated.

Ventricular tachycardia can be monomorphic (see Fig. 3.6) or polymorphic, sustained or nonsustained. Sustained VT is defined as persisting for longer than 30 s; nonsustained has at least three or more ventricular beats but lasts less than 30 s.

The signs and symptoms of ventricular dysrhythmia range from palpitations, diaphoresis, dizziness, lightheadedness, shortness of breath, chest pain, pre-syncope, syncope, and sudden cardiac death. Some patients may be completely asymptomatic. A complete history and physical exam should be performed on all patients with ventricular dysrhythmias. The patient should be questioned about a family history of sudden cardiac death and evaluated for risk factors of coronary artery disease.

Ventricular tachycardia is a wide complex rhythm that must be distinguished from supraventricular tachycardia with aberrant conduction. Clues that suggest a ventricular origin include AV dissociation, fusion beats (which result from simultaneous

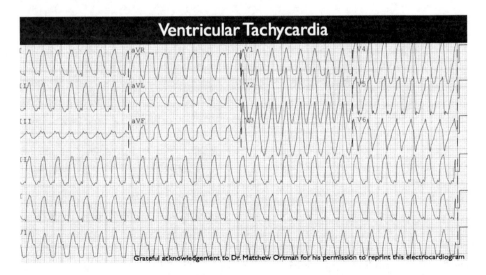

**Fig. 3.6** Ventricular tachycardia. ECG courtesy of Matthew Ortman, MD

activation of two foci, one ventricular and one supraventricular), and capture beats (beats that capture the ventricle and are conducted with a narrow complex, ruling out fixed bundle branch block), as well as severe left axis deviation (−60 to 120°). A more systematic approach to distinguish VT from a wide complex supraventricular tachycardia was outlined by Brugada [36]. The diagnosis is VT If there is absence of the RS complex in all precordial leads, R to S interval is greater than 100 ms in one precordial lead, AV dissociation, or characteristic morphology in leads $V_1$, $V_2$ and $V_6$, the diagnosis is ventricular tachycardia. If not, the arrhythmia is most likely supraventricular tachycardia with aberrant conduction.

Sustained monomorphic VT is a reentrant rhythm most commonly occurring more than 48 h after a myocardial infarction, or in the setting of cardiomyopathy. Initial management of sustained monomorphic VT with a history of structural heart disease depends on its rate, duration, and hemodynamic status. Unstable VT is an indication for prompt defibrillation. Hemodynamically stable patients with a risk of imminent circulatory collapse may be treated with an antiarrhythmic such as IV amiodarone. Current ACLS guidelines consider lidocaine and IV procainamide alternative choices. If the arrhythmia recurs, intravenous antiarrhythmic drug therapy, with either amiodarone, lidocaine, or procainamide should be initiated.

Enthusiasm for the use of chronic antiarrhythmic agents to prevent ventricular arrhythmias was considerably dampened after the Cardiac Arrhythmia Suppression Trial [37], which showed an increase in mortality in patients receiving flecainide or encainide in patients with coronary artery disease [17]. There has been concern that other antiarrhythmic agents could have the same proarrhythmic effects. Available data suggest that amiodarone and sotalol are the most effective antiarrhythmic drugs for preventing sustained ventricular tachycardia.

Clinical trials comparing insertion of automated implantable cardioverter defibrillators (AICD) to antiarrhythmic drug therapy have generally shown a benefit for AICD placement. In high-risk patients (non-sustained VT, prior Q-wave myocardial infarction, ejection fraction ≤35%, inducible sustained VT not suppressed by procainamide at electrophysiological study), the MADIT [38] study showed significantly improved survival with AICD compared to conventional medical therapy [38]. Similarly, the AVID [39] Study showed that patients resuscitated from ventricular fibrillation or with hemodynamically significant VT with EF ≤40% had improved survival with AICD compared to antiarrhythmic therapy (amiodarone in more than 80%) [39].

AICD placement appears to be effective as primary prevention as well. The MADIT-II trial demonstrated that prophylactic placement of an implantable cardioverter defibrillator (ICD) in patients with LVEF ≤30% after myocardial infarction improved survival [40]. The timing of ICD implantation however is uncertain. In the recent Defibrillator in Acute Myocardial Infarction Trial (DINAMIT) study, placement of an ICD immediately after a myocardial infarction did not reduce all-cause mortality [41], and analysis of MADIT-II demonstrated that patients with a remote myocardial infarction (at least 18 months previous) benefited greatly from the ICD, whereas, those with a more recent myocardial infarction (less than 18 months) did not [42]. Data from the SCD-Heft (Sudden Cardiac Death-Heart Failure) trial also showed a survival benefit in patients with either an ischemic or a non-ischemic cardiomyopathy and EF <35% after implantation of an AICD compared to amiodarone [43]. Due to the outcomes of these trials, implantable defibrillators are recommended for survivors of sudden cardiac death and patients with a previous myocardial infarction and LV ejection fractions of less than 35%.

The challenge in selecting patients for AICD implantation is that identification of the highest risk subgroups leads to very cost-effective use of devices but identifies only a small proportion of the total of 300,000 sudden cardiac deaths that occur annually in the United States [37]. Improvement in risk stratification techniques and strategies to consider costs and benefits in the general population is driving the evolution of AICD use in the community.

## Torsade de Pointes

Torsade de pointes is a syndrome consisting of polymorphic VT with QT prolongation. Polymorphic VT without QT prolongation most commonly occurs in the setting of acute myocardial ischemia. Although polymorphic VT is often faster than sustained monomorphic VT and thus can lead to hemodynamic instability, many episodes of polymorphic VT terminate spontaneously. Initial management for polymorphic VT without QT prolongation is similar to that for monomorphic VT, with defibrillation and antiarrhythmic drugs [44].

Torsade de pointes can occur in the absence of structural heart disease. Acquired QT prolongation is most often caused by drugs, including type I and type III antiarrhythmic agents, tricyclic antidepressants, phenothiazines, nonsedating antihistamines, erythromycin, pentamidine, and azole antifungal agents. QT prolongation may also be caused by electrolyte abnormalities, especially hypomagnesemia, and exacerbated by other conditions such as hypothyroidism, cerebrovascular accident, and liquid protein diets [45].

Torsade de pointes is triggered by early afterdepolarizations, oscillations in the membrane potential that occur during prolonged repolarization, usually in the setting of an accumulation of intracellular positive ions. This abnormality can occur from malfunctioning ion channels, electrolyte disruptions or by medications, and may be exacerbated by increased sympathetic activity. The early afterdepolarizations depolarize nearby cell membranes, which can result in action potentials, initiating polymorphic VT.

The EKG of torsade de pointes will show a beat-to-beat change in the QRS axis, irregular RR intervals, and a heart rate ranging from 160 to 250 beats/min (see Fig. 3.7). A pause may be seen before the onset of Torsade. Ventricular bigeminy in a patient with a long QT interval may be a sign of impending Torsade. On the resting EKG, The QT interval varies inversely with the heart rate and therefore must be corrected, usually using Bazett's formula, in which the corrected QT interval (QTc) is the QT interval divided by the square root of the RR interval in msec. A QTc of greater than 0.44 s in men and greater than 0.45 s in women is considered prolonged.

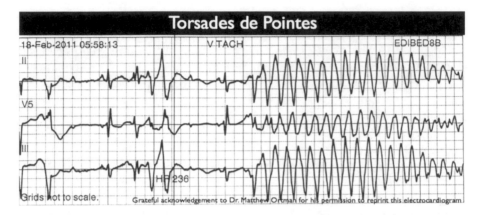

**Fig. 3.7** Torsades de pointes. Note initiation after a long R–R interval followed by a shorter one. ECG courtesy of Matthew Ortman, MD

Empiric magnesium (2 g IV over 1–2 min) should be given to all patients with suspected torsade de pointes, since the risk is low and the potential benefits high. Since the length of the QT interval is affected by the RR interval, in patients with acquired QT prolongation and torsade de pointes, use of isoproterenol or temporary pacing to increase the heart rate can be effective [46]. Nonsynchronized electrical defibrillation may be required in hemodynamically unstable patients.

## Long QT Syndrome

Congenital long QT (LQT) syndrome is a disorder of ventricular repolarization characterized by a prolonged QT interval. This prolongation of the QT interval predisposes the patient to torsade de pointes, ventricular fibrillation and sudden cardiac death. Forms of congenital long QT syndrome include Jervell and Lange-Nielsen syndrome, which is associated with sensorineural deafness, and Romano-Ward syndrome. Genes responsible for long QT syndrome have been identified and the syndrome classified into subtypes according to mutation. Of the two most common mutations, LQT type 1 is associated with mutations in KVLQT1, an outward-rectifying cardiac potassium channel protein, LQT type 2 with mutations in the human ether-related-a-go-go (HERG) gene, another component of the outward-rectifying potassium channel, and LQT type 3 with mutations in the cardiac sodium channel gene SCN5A. This is important because these three subtypes have different arrhythmic triggers and respond differently to medications. Long QT syndrome is perhaps the best example of the use of genotyping to guide prognosis and therapy in current cardiologic practice.

The signs and symptoms of congenital LQTS occur during childhood or adolescence. Syncope or cardiac arrest during physical exertion or emotional stress may be the first presenting symptom. Arrhythmic events in patients with LQT1 are most often related to exercise, and also with swimming. Events triggered by auditory stimuli, such as alarm clocks and telephones, are most typically seen in patients with LQT2. Patients with LQT3 are at highest risk of events when at rest or asleep. The clinical course of LQTS is also influenced by genotype; patients with LQT1 tend to have the earliest events and a worse prognosis, and those with LQT3 have a later onset and a lower overall event rate. There is also a difference in clinical course with different mutations within one subtype.

The mainstay of pharmacologic therapy for congenital long QT syndrome is beta blockade, titrated to blunt the maximum heart rate achieved by exertion. Competitive sports should be avoided. The efficacy of beta blockers varies with genotype; they are most effective in patients with LQT1, and least effective in patients with LQT3. Left cardiac sympathetic denervation is occasionally performed to prevent cardiac events. Cardiac pacing has been employed in patients who remain symptomatic despite medical therapy, and may be especially useful in patients with LQT3. AICD implantation is recommended in patients who have recurrent syncope, sustained ventricular arrhythmias, or sudden cardiac death despite drug therapy [47, 48].

## Arrhythmogenic Right Ventricular Dysplasia

Arrhythmogenic right ventricular dysplasia (ARVD) is a myocardial disorder in which there is replacement of the right ventricle myocardium with fatty or fibrofatty tissue, with the potential for a reentrant ventricular tachycardia and sudden death. ARVD occurs in families, with both an autosomal dominant and autosomal recessive form. A familial form of ARVD accompanied by hyperkeratosis and woolly hair with autosomal recessive inheritance was identified on a Greek island and termed Naxos disease.

The clinical manifestations include palpitations, dizziness, syncope, right-sided heart failure, sustained or nonsustained monomorphic VT and sudden cardiac death. The EKG is characteristic, including a prolonged QRS complex with a right bundle branch pattern, epsilon wave (electric potentials after the end of the QRS complex), and T wave inversions in leads $V_1$–$V_3$. Diagnostic testing includes echocardiography, signal-averaged electrocardiography, and MRI, which is the best method to demonstrate fatty infiltration of the right ventricular myocardium. Signal-averaged electrocardiography may be used to screen family members.

Both ventricular tachycardia and sudden death can be exercise-induced, possibly due to RV stress and catecholamine stimulation, so patients with ARVD should not participate in competitive sports. Therapy should be aimed at suppression of arrhythmias. Sotalol is the most effective antiarrhythmic medication for suppressing ventricular arrhythmias in ARVD. Amiodarone is the second choice. Implantable defibrillators are indicated (Class I) for symptomatic patients and survivors of sudden cardiac death, and may be considered (Class IIa) for secondary prevention and a Class IIa for primary prevention of ventricular tachycardia in ARVD [49].

Ablation of arrhythmic foci has been undertaken, but ARVD tends to progress, and so this therapy is usually reserved for patients with non-life threatening but symptomatic tachyarrhythmias who are intolerant of antiarrhythmic drugs.

## Brugada Syndrome

Brugada syndrome is a rare genetic disease that is characterized by ST elevation unrelated to electrolyte disorders or coronary ischemia. Brugada syndrome can cause sudden cardiac death from ventricular fibrillation in individuals with structurally normal hearts. The EKG findings are distinctive, and include a pseudo-right bundle branch block pattern with ST elevation in leads $V_1$–$V_3$. Cases of Brugada syndrome have now been linked with mutations in the cardiac sodium channel gene, SCN5A [50]. There is some suggestion that Brugada syndrome may be an early manifestation of arrhythmogenic right ventricular dysplasia, but this is uncertain.

The diagnosis of Brugada syndrome relies upon the ECG findings and the clinical presentation. The diagnosis of Brugada syndrome should be considered if the patient has coved type ST segment elevation in more than one precordial lead and one of the following: documented ventricular fibrillation; self-terminating polymorphic ventricular tachycardia; a family history of sudden cardiac death at age less than 45 years old; coved ST segment elevation in family members; electrophysiologic inducibility; syncope; and nocturnal agonal respiration [51]. A patient with ECG findings without clinical manifestations is defined as having Brugada pattern [51].

There are no well established pharmacologic therapies. Beta blockers and amiodarone have not been shown to be beneficial. There is some suggestion that quinidine may be useful [52].

Implantation of an AICD is the only currently proven therapy to prevent sudden death, and is recommended in patients with syncope, symptomatic VT, or a prior history of aborted sudden cardiac death [47, 49]. What to do with asymptomatic patients is less certain. Stratification by electrophysiologic testing, with AICD implantation in patients with inducible VT, has been advocated [48].

## Bradycardias

### Sinus Node Dysfunction

Bradycardias associated with sinus node dysfunction include sinus bradycardia, sinus pause, sinoatrial block, and sinus arrest. These disturbances often result from increased vagal tone [53]. If bradycardia is transient and not associated with hemodynamic compromise, no therapy is necessary. If bradycardia is sustained or compromises end-organ perfusion, therapy with antimuscarinic agents such as atropine, or beta agonists such as ephedrine may be initiated. Transcutaneous or transvenous pacing may be necessary in some cases.

Patients with a combination of bradycardia with paroxysmal atrial tachycardias due to preexisting conduction system disease can be challenging to manage pharmacologically. In these cases, insertion of a temporary pacemaker may allow the administration of rate lowering agents.

## Heart Block

The most common cause of acquired chronic atrioventricular (AV) heart block is fibrosis of the conducting system. Although preexisting conduction system disease is a risk factor for the development of complete heart block, no single laboratory or clinical variable identifies patients at risk for progression to high degree AV block [47]. In first-degree AV block there is prolongation of conduction time of the atrial impulses to the ventricles, with PR intervals greater than 200 ms. In second-degree AV block, conducted atrial beats are interspersed with nonconducted beats. Second-degree AV block is divided into Mobitz type I (Wenckebach) (see Fig. 3.8) and Mobitz Type II block (see Fig. 3.9). In Mobitz I block, the PR interval lengthens progressively until the p-wave fails to conduct. In most cases the block occurs at the AV node. Mobitz I block can occur in healthy individuals, the elderly and in patients with underlying heart disease. In Mobitz type II AV block, the PR interval remains constant until a p-wave fails to conduct. Mobitz II block occurs below the AV node, and thus is more dangerous since it is much more likely to progress to complete

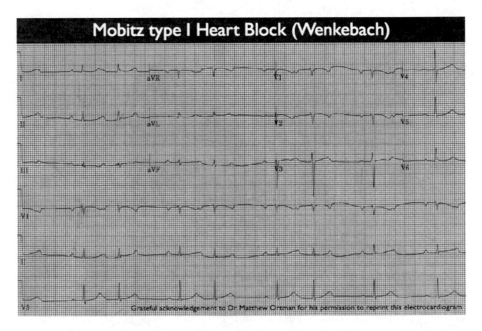

**Fig. 3.8** Mobitz type I second degree (Wenckebach) heart block. The PR interval of the first conducted beat after the pause is shorter than the PR interval of the last conducted beat before the pause. ECG courtesy of Matthew Ortman, MD

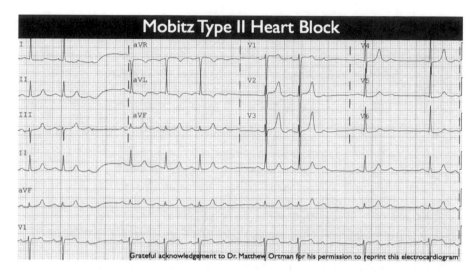

**Fig. 3.9** Mobitz type II second degree heart block. All of the conducted PR intervals are the same. ECG courtesy of Matthew Ortman, MD

heart block. In third-degree AV block, none of the atrial impulses are conducted to the ventricles. The escape rhythm, whether junctional or ventricular, is generally regular (see Fig. 3.10).

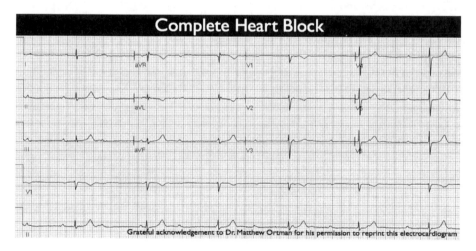

**Fig. 3.10** Complete heart block. ECG Courtesy of Matthew Ortman, MD

Patients with AV block may be asymptomatic, but may experience dizziness or syncope as a consequence of decreased cardiac output. AV block is most commonly caused by AV nodal conduction disease, but AV nodal blocking agents need to be ruled out as causative agents. Any medications that affect conduction through the AV node should be decreased or discontinued if possible.

Recommendations for pacemaker implantation differ a bit among societies, but in general are predicated on symptoms and the potential for progression to higher degrees of heart block. A pacemaker is generally not recommended in most cases of first-degree AV block, although it may be considered in patients with marked PR prolongation (>300 ms) and LV dysfunction with heart failure symptoms [47]. In patients with second or third degree block and either symptomatic bradycardia or congestive heart failure is a Class I indication (general agreement that a treatment is beneficial) for insertion of a pacemaker [47]. The ACC/AHA/NASPE have given permanent pacing for asymptomatic patients with Mobitz type II AV block a Class IIa recommendation (conflicting evidence, but weight of evidence favors usefulness) [47]. Permanent pacing was given a Class I indication for all patients with third degree or advanced heart block and either symptomatic bradycardia, pauses greater than 3 s, or escape rates less than 40 beats/min. A Class IIa recommendation for permanent pacing was given for patients with asymptomatic third-degree AV block [47].

Pacemaker implantation is also indicated in patients who have bradycardia-tachycardia ("sick sinus") syndrome, and other arrhythmias or medical conditions that require drugs that result in symptomatic bradycardia [47]. Pacing may also be considered for patients with an inadequate chronotropic response to exercise.

Conduction abnormalities are common complications of acute myocardial infarctions. These can be transient or permanent. Conduction abnormalities associated with an acute inferior myocardial infarction are usually result from AV nodal ischemia, are transient, and carry with a low mortality rate. Conduction abnormalities in association with an acute anterior myocardial infarction, however, represent extensive necrosis of the infranodal conduction system and the myocardium, and are associated with high in-hospital mortality [54]. The ACC/AHA/NASPE recommended guidelines for permanent and temporary implantation of pacemakers in patients with an acute myocardial infarction are shown in Tables 3.2 and 3.3.

**Table 3.2** Recommendations for permanent pacing after the acute phase of myocardial infarction (Adapted from Gregoratos et al. [47])

---

Class I

Persistent second-degree AV block in the His–Purkinje system with bilateral bundle branch block or complete heart block after acute myocardial infarction

Transient advanced (second or third degree) infranodal AV block and associated bundle-branch block. If the site of block is uncertain, an electrophysiologic study may be necessary

Persistent and symptomatic second or third degree AV block

Class IIb

Persistent second or third degree AV block at the AV node level

Class III

Transient AV block in the absence of intraventricular conduction defects

Transient AV block in the presence of isolated left anterior fascicular block

Acquired left anterior fascicular block in the absence of AV block

Persistent first-degree AV block in the presence of bundle-branch block that is old or age indeterminate

---

**Table 3.3** Recommendations for temporary transvenous pacing after an acute myocardial infarction (Adapted from Ryan et al. [55])

Class I
  Asystole
  Symptomatic bradycardia
  Bilateral bundle branch block (alternating BBB or RBBB with alternating LAFB/LPFB, any age)
  New or indeterminate-age bifascicular block (RBBB with LAFB or LPFB, or LBBB) with
      first-degree AV block
  Mobitz type II second-degree AV block

Class IIa
  RBBB and LAFB or LPFB (new or indeterminate)
  RBBB with first-degree AV block
  LBBB, new or indeterminate
  Incessant VT, for atrial or ventricular overdrive pacing
  Recurrent sinus pauses (greater than 3 s) not responsive to atropine.

Class IIB
  Bifascicular block of indeterminate age
  New or age-indeterminate isolated RBBB

Class III
  First degree heart block
  Type I second-degree AV block with normal hemodynamics
  Accelerated idioventricular rhythm
  BBB or fascicular block known to exist before AMI

*RBBB* right bundle branch block; *LBBB* left bundle branch block; *LAFB* left anterior fascicular block; *LPFV* left posterior fascicular block; *AMI* acute myocardial infarction

# References

1. Marriott HJL. Practical electrocardiography. Baltimore: Williams & Wilkins; 1988.
2. Go AS, Hylek EM, Phillips KA, et al. Prevalence of diagnosed atrial fibrillation in adults: national implications for rhythm management and stroke prevention: the anticoagulation and risk factors in atrial fibrillation (ATRIA) study. JAMA. 2001;285:2370–5.
3. Rathore SS, Berger AK, Weinfurt KP, et al. Acute myocardial infarction complicated by atrial fibrillation in the elderly: prevalence and outcomes. Circulation. 2000;101:969–74.
4. Fuster V, Ryden LE, Asinger RW, et al. ACC/AHA/ESC guidelines for the management of patients with atrial fibrillation: executive summary. A report of the American College of Cardiology/American Heart Association Task Force on Practice Guidelines and the European Society of Cardiology Committee for Practice Guidelines and Policy Conferences (Committee to Develop Guidelines for the Management of Patients With Atrial Fibrillation): developed in Collaboration With the North American Society of Pacing and Electrophysiology. J Am Coll Cardiol. 2001;38:1231–66.
5. Jalife J. Experimental and clinical AF mechanisms: bridging the divide. J Interv Card Electrophysiol. 2003;9:85–92.
6. Haissaguerre M, Jais P, Shah DC, et al. Spontaneous initiation of atrial fibrillation by ectopic beats originating in the pulmonary veins. N Engl J Med. 1998;339:659–66.
7. Chen SA, Tai CT, Yu WC, et al. Right atrial focal atrial fibrillation: electrophysiologic characteristics and radiofrequency catheter ablation. J Cardiovasc Electrophysiol. 1999;10:328–35.
8. Jais P, Haissaguerre M, Shah DC, et al. A focal source of atrial fibrillation treated by discrete radiofrequency ablation. Circulation. 1997;95:572–6.

9. Wyse DG, Waldo AL, DiMarco JP, et al. A comparison of rate control and rhythm control in patients with atrial fibrillation. N Engl J Med. 2002;347:1825–33.

10. Van Gelder IC, Hagens VE, Bosker HA, et al. A comparison of rate control and rhythm control in patients with recurrent persistent atrial fibrillation. N Engl J Med. 2002;347:1834–40.

11. Hohnloser SH, Kuck KH, Lilienthal J. Rhythm or rate control in atrial fibrillation – pharmacological intervention in atrial fibrillation (PIAF): a randomised trial. Lancet. 2000;356: 1789–94.

12. Carlsson J, Miketic S, Windeler J, et al. Randomized trial of rate-control versus rhythm-control in persistent atrial fibrillation: the strategies of treatment of atrial fibrillation (STAF) study. J Am Coll Cardiol. 2003;41:1690–6.

13. Snow V, Weiss KB, LeFevre M, et al. Management of newly detected atrial fibrillation: a clinical practice guideline from the American Academy of Family Physicians and the American College of Physicians. Ann Intern Med. 2003;139:1009–17.

14. Manning WJ, Silverman DI, Gordon SPF, Krumholz HM, Douglas PS. Conversion from atrial fibrillation without prolonged anticoagulation with use of transesophageal echocardiography to exclude the presence of atrial thrombi. N Engl J Med. 1993;328:750–5.

15. Goldschlager N, Epstein AE, Naccarelli G, Olshansky B, Singh B. Practical guidelines for clinicians who treat patients with amiodarone. Practice guidelines subcommittee, North American Society of pacing and electrophysiology. Arch Intern Med. 2000;160:1741–8.

16. Cardiac Arrhythmia Suppression Trial II Investigators. Effect of the antiarrhythmic agent moricizine on survival after myocardial infarction. N Engl J Med. 1992;327:227–33.

17. Echt DS, Liebson PR, Mitchell LB, et al. Mortality and morbidity in patients receiving encainide, flecainide, or placebo. The Cardiac Arrhythmia Suppression Trial. N Engl J Med. 1991; 324:781–8.

18. Wolf PA, Dawber TR, Thomas Jr HE, Kannel WB. Epidemiologic assessment of chronic atrial fibrillation and risk of stroke: the Framingham study. Neurology. 1978;28:973–7.

19. Atrial Fibrillation Investigators. Risk factors for stroke and efficacy of antithrombotic therapy in atrial fibrillation. Analysis of pooled data from five randomized controlled trials. Arch Intern Med. 1994;154:1449–57.

20. Hart RG, Pearce LA, McBride R, Rothbart RM, Asinger RW. Factors associated with ischemic stroke during aspirin therapy in atrial fibrillation: analysis of 2012 participants in the SPAF I-III clinical trials. The Stroke Prevention in Atrial Fibrillation (SPAF) Investigators. Stroke. 1999;30:1223–9.

21. Gage BF, Waterman AD, Shannon W, Boechler M, Rich MW, Radford MJ. Validation of clinical classification schemes for predicting stroke: results from the National Registry of Atrial Fibrillation. JAMA. 2001;285:2864–70.

22. Wann LS, Curtis AB, Ellenbogen KA, et al. ACCF/AHA/HRS Focused Update on the management of patients with atrial fibrillation (update on Dabigatran): a report of the American College of Cardiology Foundation Foundation/American Heart Association Task Force on practice guidelines. J Am Coll Cardiol. 2011;57:1330–7.

23. Connolly SJ, Ezekowitz MD, Yusuf S, et al. Dabigatran versus warfarin in patients with atrial fibrillation. N Engl J Med. 2009;361:1139–51.

24. Wood MA, Brown-Mahoney C, Kay GN, Ellenbogen KA. Clinical outcomes after ablation and pacing therapy for atrial fibrillation: a meta-analysis. Circulation. 2000;101:1138–44.

25. Bauernfeind RA, Amat YLF, Dhingra RC, Kehoe R, Wyndham C, Rosen KM. Chronic nonparoxysmal sinus tachycardia in otherwise healthy persons. Ann Intern Med. 1979;91:702–10.

26. Blomstrom-Lundqvist C, Scheinman MM, Aliot EM, et al. ACC/AHA/ESC guidelines for the management of patients with supraventricular arrhythmias – executive summary: a report of the American College of Cardiology/American Heart Association Task Force on Practice Guidelines and the European Society of Cardiology Committee for Practice Guidelines (Writing Committee to Develop Guidelines for the Management of Patients With Supraventricular Arrhythmias). Circulation. 2003;108:1871–909.

27. McCord J, Borzak S. Multifocal atrial tachycardia. Chest. 1998;113:203–9.

28. Levine JH, Michael JR, Guarnieri T. Treatment of multifocal atrial tachycardia with vera-pamil. N Engl J Med. 1985;312:21–5.
29. Kastor J. Arrhythmias. Philadelphia: WB Saunders; 1994.
30. Mazgalev TN, Tchou PJ. Surface potentials from the region of the atrioventricular node and their relation to dual pathway electrophysiology. Circulation. 2000;101:2110–7.
31. Scheinman MM, Huang S. The 1998 NASPE prospective catheter ablation registry. Pacing Clin Electrophysiol. 2000;23:1020–8.
32. Campbell RW, Smith RA, Gallagher JJ, Pritchett EL, Wallace AG. Atrial fibrillation in the preexcitation syndrome. Am J Cardiol. 1977;40:514–20.
33. Jackman WM, Wang XZ, Friday KJ, et al. Catheter ablation of accessory atrioventricular pathways (Wolff-Parkinson-White syndrome) by radiofrequency current. N Engl J Med. 1991;324:1605–11.
34. Wang L, Yao R. Radiofrequency catheter ablation of accessory pathway-mediated tachycardia is a safe and effective long-term therapy. Arch Med Res. 2003;34:394–8.
35. Lee KL, Chun HM, Liem LB, Sung RJ. Effect of adenosine and verapamil in catecholamine-induced accelerated atrioventricular junctional rhythm: insights into the underlying mecha-nism. Pacing Clin Electrophysiol. 1999;22:866–70.
36. Brugada P, Brugada J, Mont L, Smeets J, Andries EW. A new approach to the differential diagnosis of a regular tachycardia with a wide QRS complex. Circulation. 1991;83:1649–59.
37. Myerburg RJ, Mitrani R, Interian Jr A, Castellanos A. Interpretation of outcomes of antiar-rhythmic clinical trials: design features and population impact. Circulation. 1998;97:1514–21.
38. Moss AJ, Hall WJ, Cannom DS, et al. Improved survival with an implanted defibrillator in patients with coronary disease at high risk for ventricular arrhythmia. N Engl J Med. 1996;335:1933–40.
39. Antiarrhythmics Versus Implantable Defibrillators (AVID) Investigators. A comparison of antiarrhythmic-drug therapy with implantable defibrillators in patients resuscitated from near-fatal ventricular arrhythmias. The Antiarrhythmics versus Implantable Defibrillators (AVID) Investigators. N Engl J Med. 1997;337:1576–83.
40. Moss AJ, Zareba W, Hall WJ, et al. Prophylactic implantation of a defibrillator in patients with myocardial infarction and reduced ejection fraction. N Engl J Med. 2002;346:877–83.
41. Hohnloser SH, Kuck KH, Dorian P, et al. Prophylactic use of an implantable cardioverter-defibrillator after acute myocardial infarction. N Engl J Med. 2004;351:2481–8.
42. Greenberg H, Case RB, Moss AJ, Brown MW, Carroll ER, Andrews ML. Analysis of mortal-ity events in the Multicenter Automatic Defibrillator Implantation Trial (MADIT-II). J Am Coll Cardiol. 2004;43:1459–65.
43. Bardy GH, Lee KL, Mark DB, et al. Amiodarone or an implantable cardioverter-defibrillator for congestive heart failure. N Engl J Med. 2005;352:225–37.
44. Grogin HR, Scheinman M. Evaluation and management of patients with polymorphic ventricular tachycardia. Cardiol Clin. 1993;11:39–54.
45. Napolitano C, Priori SG, Schwartz PJ. Torsade de pointes. Mechanisms and management. Drugs. 1994;47:51–65.
46. Roden DM. Torsade de pointes. Clin Cardiol. 1993;16:683–6.
47. Gregoratos G, Cheitlin MD, Conill A, et al. ACC/AHA Guidelines for Implantation of Cardiac Pacemakers and Antiarrhythmia Devices: Executive Summary – a report of the American College of Cardiology/American Heart Association Task Force on Practice Guidelines (Committee on Pacemaker Implantation). Circulation. 1998;97:1325–35.
48. Antzelevitch C, Brugada P, Borggrefe M, et al. Brugada syndrome: report of the second consensus conference. Hear Rhythm. 2005;2:429–40.
49. Priori SG, Aliot E, Blomstrom-Lundqvist C, et al. Task force on sudden cardiac death of the European Society of cardiology. Eur Heart J. 2001;22:1374–450.
50. Chen Q, Kirsch GE, Zhang D, et al. Genetic basis and molecular mechanism for idiopathic ventricular fibrillation. Nature. 1998;392:293–6.

51. Wilde AA, Antzelevitch C, Borggrefe M, et al. Proposed diagnostic criteria for the Brugada syndrome. Eur Heart J. 2002;23:1648–54.
52. Belhassen B, Glick A, Viskin S. Efficacy of quinidine in high-risk patients with Brugada syndrome. Circulation. 2004;110:1731–7.
53. Atlee JL. Perioperative cardiac dysrhythmias: diagnosis and management. Anesthesiology. 1997;86:1397–424.
54. Hindman MC, Wagner GS, Jaro M, et al. The clinical significance of bundle branch block complicating acute myocardial infarction. Indications for temporary and permanent pacemaker insertion. Circulation. 1978;58:689–99.
55. Ryan TJ, Antman EM, Books NH, et al. 1999 Update: ACC/AHA guidelines for the management of patients with acute myocardial infarction: Executive summary and recommendation. A report of the American college of Cardiology/American Heart Association Task Force on Practice Guidelines (Committee on Management of Acute Myocardial Infarction). Circulation. 1999;100:1016.

# Chapter 4
# Hypertension

## Etiology and Pathophysiology

Hypertension is highly prevalent in the United States and worldwide, and it is a major risk factor for coronary artery disease, stroke, heart failure, renal disease, and cardiovascular events [1]. The prevalence of hypertension increases with age. The Framingham Heart Study reported a 90% lifetime risk for developing hypertension in patients who are normotensive at the age of 50 [2]. The risk of cardiovascular disease doubles with each increment of 20/10 mmHg above 115/75 [3]. Systolic hypertension is now considered a more important risk factor than diastolic pressure [4, 5].

An estimated 50 million Americans have high blood pressure, but awareness, treatment, and control is still poor, especially in the elderly [6]. A national health survey performed from 1988 to 1991 [7], and repeated from 1999 to 2000 found that the prevalence of hypertension has increased from 20 to 27% over the past decade [6]. The 1999–2000 survey found that one third of hypertensive patients were not aware of their disease, less than two-thirds adopted lifestyle modification or took medication to lower their blood pressure, and only 31% were at their blood pressure goal [6]. It is little consolation that international blood pressure control rates were no better. Between 2004 and 2008, there was a (29.4%) reduction in the rate of uncontrolled hypertension, indicating that progress has been made toward the American Heart Association's (AHA) Impact 2010 goals for CHD and stroke [8]. The most recent AHA Impact 2020 goals call for even greater reductions in the prevalence of hypertension along with the other major risk factor for vascular disease (goal untreated BP <120/80 mmHg).

Although hypertension is initiated by pathophysiologic factors that increase peripheral resistance or cardiac output, long-standing hypertension, results in stiffening of conduit arteries, and this stiffening may be a more important determinant of cardiovascular risk than the etiology of hypertension in itself [9]. Increased stiffness of large arteries leads to early wave reflection that impacts the heart during systole rather than diastole, increasing peak systolic pressure and myocardial

S. Hollenberg and S. Heitner, *Cardiology in Family Practice: A Practical Guide*, Current Clinical Practice 1, DOI 10.1007/978-1-61779-385-1_4, © Springer Science+Business Media, LLC 2012

oxygen demand, while decreasing diastolic pressure and myocardial blood supply [10]. Early wave reflection increases pulse pressure, and a widened pulse pressure has also been shown to be independently associated with subsequent myocardial infarction and other cardiovascular events [11].

About 90% of hypertension is characterized as essential, or idiopathic. Important secondary causes of hypertension include renal artery stenosis, hyperaldosteronism, renal parenchymal disease, pheochromocytoma, coarctation of the aorta, and illicit drugs. Hypertension is a heterogeneous disorder in which the different predisposing factors operate in different patients. The blood pressure in any individual depends on an interaction between expression of genes that influence blood pressure and a variety of environmental factors including diet, alcohol intake, age, socioeconomic status, lifestyle, and stress.

## Diagnosis

The classification of hypertension has recently been simplified to improve recognition of hypertension by both patients and health care providers. The classifications have been tied to treatment algorithms in the recommendations of the 7th Joint National Committee (JNC 7) [12].

The classification of blood pressure (outlined in Table 4.1) is based on the average of two or more properly measured blood pressure readings on two separate occasions. The category of prehypertension is not intended to indicate a disease state, but rather to identify individuals at high risk of developing hypertension, and to target those individuals for preventive efforts [12].

**Table 4.1** Classification of blood pressure for adults (Adapted from Chobanian et al. [12])

| BP classification | Systolic blood pressure (mmHg) | Diastolic blood pressure (mmHg) |
| --- | --- | --- |
| Normal | <120 | and <80 |
| Prehypertension | 120–139 | or 80–89 |
| Stage 1 hypertension | 140–159 | or 90–99 |
| Stage 2 hypertension | >160 | or >100 |

Once a patient is determined to be either prehypertensive or hypertensive, a thorough assessment of risk factors, possible secondary causes, and therapeutic targets should be initiated [12]. The physician should inquire about cigarette smoking, obesity, family history of cardiovascular disease, alcohol use, physical activity, and other cardiovascular risk factors (hyperlipidemia, diabetes, sedentary lifestyle). Factors that may point to secondary causes of hypertension, particularly, use of prescription or nonprescription drugs, merit scrutiny.

A complete physical exam and diagnostic tests should be performed to evaluate for signs of end organ damage and secondary causes of hypertension. Blood pressure should be obtained in both arms. A funduscopic exam should be performed to evaluate for papilledema, retinal hemorrhage or exudates, arterio-venous nicking or arteriolar narrowing. The cardiothoracic exam should include evaluation of jugular venous pressure, heart size, and auscultation for murmurs, gallops, rales, or rhonchi. The carotid, subclavian, femoral, and renal arteries should be auscultated for bruits. The abdomen should be examined for renal masses or aortic or renal artery bruits, the extremities examined for edema, and peripheral pulses palpated. The diagnostic workup should include an electrocardiogram, complete blood count, chemistry panel with attention to electrolytes, BUN, creatinine, glucose, and calcium, urinalysis, and a fasting lipid profile. Echocardiography is more sensitive for left ventricular hypertrophy than EKG, and is important at prognostication [13].

## Therapy

Lifestyle modifications alone have been shown to reduce blood pressure and cardiovascular disease complications. Lifestyle modifications include weight reduction, the Dietary Approaches to Stop Hypertension (DASH) diet (rich in fruits, vegetables, grains, low-fat dairy products, fish, and poultry), limiting sodium to <2.4 g/day, regular exercise and moderation of alcohol intake. The DASH trial showed that adherence to the DASH diet lowered systolic blood pressure by 5.5 mmHg and diastolic blood pressure by 3.0 mmHg [14]. This trial also showed a reduction in blood pressure of normotensive subjects participating in the study. The DASH-Sodium trial added low salt intake (3 g/day compared to the average intake of 9 g in developed countries) to the DASH diet, resulted in a reduction in systolic BP by 7.1 mmHg [15]. Based on these results, therapeutic lifestyle modification forms an important cornerstone in maintaining cardiovascular health for all people, but especially for those who fall either into the prehypertensive or hypertensive categories.

The approach recommended in the Joint National Committee on Prevention, Detection, Evaluation, and Treatment of High Blood Pressure (JNC 7) bases therapeutic recommendations on both the degree of hypertension and the underlying risk of cardiovascular disease. Patients are divided into those with uncomplicated hypertension and those with high-risk conditions, which are termed "compelling indications" for the use of other antihypertensive drug classes (see Table 4.2).

For hypertensive patients without compelling indications, thiazide diuretics or beta blockers should be the first choice [12]. This recommendation was based largely on the outcome of the ALLHAT (Antihypertensive and Lipid-Lowering Treatment to Prevent Heart Attack) trial, which randomized, 33,357 participants over 55 with hypertension and at least one other coronary risk factor to chlorthalidone, amlodipine, or lisinopril (an arm with doxazosin was terminated prematurely due to adverse outcomes). After a mean follow-up of 4.9 years, there was no difference in either the primary outcome or all-cause mortality among treatments [16]. Compared directly, diuretics were equivalent to amlodipine, but superior to lisinopril, although this may have been due to improved blood pressure control with chlorthalidone ACE inhibitors, angiotension II blockers, calcium channel blocker and beta blockers are often necessary as additional agents in an effort to attain the goal blood pressure. The JNC 7 guidelines include a general goal of <140/90 mmHg for

**Table 4.2** Classification and management of blood pressure for adults (Adapted from Chobanian et al. [12])

| BP classification | SBP (mmHg) | DBP (mmHg) | Lifestyle modification | Drug therapy without compelling indications | Drug therapy with compelling indications |
|---|---|---|---|---|---|
| Normal | <120 | <80 | Encourage | None | Drugs for compelling indications |
| Prehypertension | 120–139 | 80–89 | Yes | None | Drugs for the compelling indications. Other antihypertensive drugs (diurectic, ACEI, ARB, BB, CCB) as needed |
| Stage 1 Hypertension | 140–159 | 90–99 | Yes | Thiazide-type diuretics for most. May consider ACEI, ARB, BB, CCB, or combination | |
| Stage 2 Hypertension | >160 | >100 | Yes | Two-drug combination for most (usually thiazide-type diurectic and ACEI or ARB or BB or CCB) | |

*SBP* systolic blood pressure; *DBP* diastolic blood pressure; *ACE* angiotensin-converting enzyme inhibitor; *ARB* angiotensin receptor blocker; *BB* beta blocker; *CCB* calcium channel blocker

blood pressure-lowering therapy in uncomplicated hypertension, while a goal of <130/80 mmHg is recommended for patients who have experienced ST- or non-ST-segment elevation MI, as well as for patients with diabetes, renal disease, or other high-risk conditions [17, 18].

More recently several studies have successfully shown a benefit for the use of fixed-dose combination therapies. The ACCOMPLISH study showed that the combination of the angiotensin inhibitor benazepril and the dihydropyridine calcium channel blocker amlodipine reduced both mortality and morbidity compared with benazapril plus hydrochlorothiazide [19, 20].

Several antihypertensive agents from different classes are often needed to bring patients to goal blood pressure. If the blood pressure is 20/10 mmHg above goal, then two drugs may be required as initial therapy, with one being a thiazide diuretic [12]. Some care should be exercised in order to avoid postural hypotension, particularly in the elderly and in patients with autonomic dysfunction. With regards to systolic hypertension in the elderly, the SHEP study demonstrated that drug therapy for isolated systolic hypertension in patients aged 60 or above was associated with a lower incidence of stroke and major cardiovascular events (relative reductions in myocardial infarction by 27%, heart failure by 55%, and stroke by 37%) [5]. The similarly designed Syst-Euro study showed that the use of a dihydropyridine calcium channel blocker was associated with a reduction in the frequency of vascular events, and, interestingly, also Alzheimer's dementia [21].

The guidelines do not specifically stipulate a lower limit to the goal for blood pressure in treating hypertension. There is, however, a direct statement that in the case of blood pressure therapy for secondary prevention of cardiovascular events, lower blood pressure is better [12]. This concept has recently been challenged by data from the ACCORD trial (which compared a systolic blood pressure target <120 mmHg with 140 mmHg) [22], and the extended follow-up of the INVEST study (targeting <130/85 vs. <140/90 mmHg) [23]. Both studies failed to show benefit in patients treated to aggressive goals. The plateau seen in benefit derived from lowering of systolic blood pressure beyond 120 mmHg or diastolic BP <80 mmHg has been termed the "J-curve". Several post-hoc analyses of large prospective studies (VALIANT, ONTARGET, and TNT) have also demonstrated the J-curve phenomenon [24–26]. The British Hypertension Society has developed a tool to guide the use of combination pharmacotherapy in hypertension and termed it the AB/CD rule. This tool provides a simple and easily applicable guide to aid the choice of agents in patients with hypertension not requiring compelling indications for specific agents in the setting of comorbidities or drug intolerances (see Fig. 4.1).

## Compelling Indications

For patients with hypertension and compelling indications, the treatment recommendations have been modified (Table 4.3). Hypertension and ischemic coronary disease are the most common causes of heart failure. Patients with heart failure must

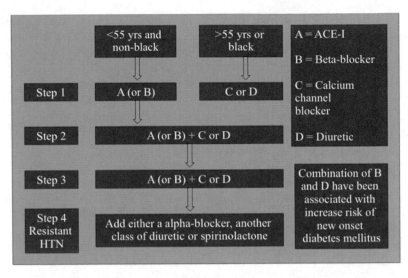

**Fig. 4.1** Recommendations for combining blood pressure lowering drugs (AB/CD rule) (Adapted from Brown et al. [46])

**Table 4.3** Guideline basis for compelling indications for individual drug classes (Adapted from Chobanian et al. [12])

| Compelling indications | Recommended drugs | | | | | |
|---|---|---|---|---|---|---|
| | Diuretic | BB | ACEI | ARB | CCB | Aldosterone antagonist |
| Heart failure | X | X | X | X | | X |
| Post-MI | | X | X | | | X |
| High CAD risk | X | X | X | | X | |
| DM | X | X | X | X | X | |
| CKD | | | X | X | | |
| CVA/TIA | X | | X | | | |

*ACEI* angiotensin-converting enzyme inhibitor; *ARB* angiotensin receptor blocker; *BB* beta blocker; *CCB* calcium channel blocker; *MI* myocardial infarction; *CAD* coronary artery disease; *DM* diabetes mellitus; *CKD* chronic kidney disease; *CVA/TIA* cerebrovascular accident/transient ischemic attack

restrict their sodium and fluid intake. In these patients, control of blood pressure is achieved with agents proven to improve outcomes in heart failure. While loop diuretics are used to relieve the symptoms of heart failure, ACE inhibitors, angiotensin receptor blockers, and beta blockers have been shown to improve morbidity and mortality in patients with systolic dysfunction [27–34]. The aldosterone antagonist spironolactone reduced the morbidity and death in patients with heart failure [35]. Along similar lines, after myocardial infarction, survival benefits have been shown with beta blockers [36, 37]. ACE inhibitors [38], and the aldosterone antagonist eplerenone [39].

Diuretics, beta blockers, ACE inhibitors, ARB, and calcium channel blockers can all be used in the treatment of hypertension in diabetics, but the initial agent should always be either an ACE inhibitor or angiotensin receptor blocker, as they have been shown to reduce the rate of progression of renal disease in diabetes [40, 41].

Blood pressure should be treated aggressively in patients with chronic kidney disease. As with diabetes, the target blood pressure may be less than 130/80, with systolic pressure being the primary target. Patients with renal insufficiency usually require more than three drugs to control their hypertension. ACE Inhibitors have been shown to be renal protective in this setting as well [42, 43].

Blood pressure control is beneficial for the prevention of stroke. The PROGRESS Trial using a combination ACE Inhibitor/thiazide diuretic drug regimen showed a significant decrease in the risk of recurrent stroke [44].

Patients should be monitored and medications adjusted monthly until the goal blood pressure is achieved. Individuals on ACE inhibitors and ARBs should have their creatinine and potassium monitored. ACE inhibitors should only be withheld if creatinine increases to greater than 50% from baseline, or potassium increases to greater than 5.6 mmol/L [45]. Once goal blood pressure is reached, the patients should follow-up every 3–6 months. Patients with compelling indications should be monitored more frequently.

Patients are considered to have resistant hypertension if the goal blood pressure is not obtained with a three-drug regimen. After investigation for secondary causes of hypertension (Table 4.4) is completed, these patients should be considered for referral to a specialist.

**Table 4.4** Secondary causes of hypertension

| |
|---|
| Drugs (non-steroidal anti-inflammatory drugs, oral contraceptives, steroids, licorice, sympathomimetics, cold remedies) |
| Renal disease |
| Renovascular disease |
| Pheochromocytoma |
| Conn's syndrome |
| Cushing's disease |
| Coarctation of the aorta |

# References

1. Messerli FH, Williams B, Ritz E. Essential hypertension. Lancet. 2007;370(9587):591–603.
2. Vasan RS et al. Residual lifetime risk for developing hypertension in middle-aged women and men: The Framingham Heart Study. JAMA. 2002;287(8):1003–10.
3. Lewington S et al. Age-specific relevance of usual blood pressure to vascular mortality: a meta-analysis of individual data for one million adults in 61 prospective studies. Lancet. 2002;360(9349):1903–13.
4. Izzo Jr JL, Levy D, Black HR. Clinical Advisory Statement. Importance of systolic blood pressure in older Americans. Hypertension. 2000;35(5):1021–4.

5.  SHEP Cooperative Research Group. Prevention of stroke by antihypertensive drug treatment in older persons with isolated systolic hypertension. Final results of the Systolic Hypertension in the Elderly Program (SHEP). JAMA. 1991;265(24):3255–64.
6.  Wang Y, Wang QJ. The prevalence of prehypertension and hypertension among US adults according to the new joint national committee guidelines: new challenges of the old problem. Arch Intern Med. 2004;164(19):2126–34.
7.  Burt VL et al. Prevalence of hypertension in the US adult population. Results from the Third National Health and Nutrition Examination Survey, 1988–1991. Hypertension. 1995;25(3): 305–13.
8.  Lloyd-Jones DM et al. Defining and setting national goals for cardiovascular health promotion and disease reduction: the American Heart Association's strategic Impact Goal through 2020 and beyond. Circulation. 2010;121(4):586–613.
9.  Franklin SS. The concept of vascular overload in hypertension. Cardiol Clin. 1995;13(4): 501–7.
10. O'Rourke MF, Kelly RF. Wave reflection in the systemic circulation and its implications in ventricular function. J Hypertens. 1993;11:327–37.
11. Madhavan S et al. Relation of pulse pressure and blood pressure reduction to the incidence of myocardial infarction. Hypertension. 1994;23:395–401.
12. Chobanian AV et al. The seventh report of the Joint National Committee on Prevention, Detection, Evaluation, and Treatment of High Blood Pressure: the JNC 7 report. JAMA. 2003;289(19):2560–72.
13. Devereux RB, Alderman MH. Role of preclinical cardiovascular disease in the evolution from risk factor exposure to development of morbid events. Circulation. 1993;88:1444–55.
14. Appel LJ et al. A clinical trial of the effects of dietary patterns on blood pressure. DASH Collaborative Research Group. N Engl J Med. 1997;336(16):1117–24.
15. Sacks FM et al. Effects on blood pressure of reduced dietary sodium and the Dietary Approaches to Stop Hypertension (DASH) diet. DASH-Sodium Collaborative Research Group. N Engl J Med. 2001;344(1):3–10.
16. Antihypertensive and Lipid-Lowering Treatment to Prevent Heart Attack Trial (ALLHAT) Collaborative Research Group. Major outcomes in high-risk hypertensive patients randomized to angiotensin-converting enzyme inhibitor or calcium channel blocker vs diuretic: the Antihypertensive and Lipid-Lowering Treatment to Prevent Heart Attack Trial (ALLHAT). JAMA. 2002;288(23):2981–97.
17. Rosendorff C et al. Treatment of hypertension in the prevention and management of ischemic heart disease: a scientific statement from the American Heart Association Council for High Blood Pressure Research and the Councils on Clinical Cardiology and Epidemiology and Prevention. Circulation. 2007;115(21):2761–88.
18. Anderson JL et al. ACC/AHA 2007 guidelines for the management of patients with unstable angina/non ST-elevation myocardial infarction: a report of the American College of Cardiology/American Heart Association Task Force on Practice Guidelines (Writing Committee to Revise the 2002 Guidelines for the Management of Patients With Unstable Angina/Non ST-Elevation Myocardial Infarction): developed in collaboration with the American College of Emergency Physicians, the Society for Cardiovascular Angiography and Interventions, and the Society of Thoracic Surgeons: endorsed by the American Association of Cardiovascular and Pulmonary Rehabilitation and the Society for Academic Emergency Medicine. Circulation. 2007;116(7):e148–304.
19. Jamerson K et al. Benazepril plus amlodipine or hydrochlorothiazide for hypertension in high-risk patients. N Engl J Med. 2008;359(23):2417–28.
20. Bakris GL et al. Renal outcomes with different fixed-dose combination therapies in patients with hypertension at high risk for cardiovascular events (ACCOMPLISH): a prespecified secondary analysis of a randomised controlled trial. Lancet. 2010;375(9721):1173–81.
21. Forette F et al. The prevention of dementia with antihypertensive treatment: new evidence from the Systolic Hypertension in Europe (Syst-Eur) study. Arch Intern Med. 2002;162(18): 2046–52.

22. Cushman WC et al. Effects of intensive blood-pressure control in type 2 diabetes mellitus. N Engl J Med. 2010;362(17):1575–85.
23. Cooper-DeHoff RM et al. Tight blood pressure control and cardiovascular outcomes among hypertensive patients with diabetes and coronary artery disease. JAMA. 2010;304(1):61–8.
24. Thune JJ et al. Effect of antecedent hypertension and follow-up blood pressure on outcomes after high-risk myocardial infarction. Hypertension. 2008;51(1):48–54.
25. Sleight P et al. Prognostic value of blood pressure in patients with high vascular risk in the Ongoing Telmisartan Alone and in combination with Ramipril Global Endpoint Trial study. J Hypertens. 2009;27(7):1360–9.
26. Bangalore S et al. J-curve revisited: an analysis of blood pressure and cardiovascular events in the Treating to New Targets (TNT) Trial. Eur Heart J. 2010;31(23):2897–908.
27. CONSENSUS Trial Study Group. Effects of enalapril on mortality in severe congestive heart failure. Results of the Cooperative North Scandanavian Enalapril Survival Study (CONSENSUS). N Engl J Med. 1987;316:1429–35.
28. SOLVD Investigators. Effect of enalapril on survival in patients with reduced left ventricular ejection fractions and congestive heart failure. N Engl J Med. 1991;325(5):293–302.
29. SOLVD Investigators. Effect of enalapril on mortality and the development of heart failure in asymptomatic patients with reduced left ventricular ejection fractions. N Engl J Med. 1992; 327(10):685–91.
30. Cohn JN, Tognoni G. A randomized trial of the angiotensin-receptor blocker valsartan in chronic heart failure. N Engl J Med. 2001;345(23):1667–75.
31. Pitt B et al. Effect of losartan compared with captopril on mortality in patients with symptomatic heart failure: randomised trial – the Losartan Heart Failure Survival Study ELITE II. Lancet. 2000;355(9215):1582–7.
32. CIBIS-II Investigators. The Cardiac Insufficiency Bisoprolol Study II (CIBIS-II): a randomised trial. Lancet. 1999;353:9–13.
33. Metoprolol CR/XL Randomised Intervention Trial in Congestive Heart Failure Investigators. Effect of metoprolol CR/XL in chronic heart failure: Metoprolol CR/XL Randomised Intervention Trial in Congestive Heart Failure (MERIT-HF). Lancet. 1999;353(9169): 2001–7.
34. Packer M et al. The effect of carvedilol on morbidity and mortality in patients with chronic heart failure. U.S. Carvedilol Heart Failure Study Group. N Engl J Med. 1996;334(21): 1349–55.
35. Pitt B et al. The effect of spironolactone on morbidity and mortality in patients with severe heart failure. Randomized Aldactone Evaluation Study Investigators. N Engl J Med. 1999;341(10):709–17.
36. Dargie HJ. Effect of carvedilol on outcome after myocardial infarction in patients with left-ventricular dysfunction: the CAPRICORN randomised trial. Lancet. 2001;357(9266): 1385–90.
37. Group International Collaborative Study. Reduction of infarct size with the early use of timolol in acute myocardial infarction. N Engl J Med. 1984;310:9–15.
38. Pfeffer MA et al. Effect of captopril on mortality and morbidity in patients with left ventricular dysfunction after myocardial infarction. Results of the Survival and Ventricular Enlargement Trial. N Engl J Med. 1992;327:669–77.
39. Pitt B et al. Eplerenone, a selective aldosterone blocker, in patients with left ventricular dysfunction after myocardial infarction. N Engl J Med. 2003;348:1309–21.
40. Jafar TH et al. Progression of chronic kidney disease: the role of blood pressure control, proteinuria, and angiotensin-converting enzyme inhibition: a patient-level meta-analysis. Ann Intern Med. 2003;139(4):244–52.
41. Brenner BM et al. Effects of losartan on renal and cardiovascular outcomes in patients with type 2 diabetes and nephropathy. N Engl J Med. 2001;345(12):861–9.
42. GISEN (Gruppo Italiano di Studi Epidemiologici in Nefrologia Group). Randomised placebo-controlled trial of effect of ramipril on decline in glomerular filtration rate and risk of terminal renal failure in proteinuric, non-diabetic nephropathy. Lancet. 1997;349(9069):1857–63.

43. Ruggenenti P et al. Renoprotective properties of ACE-inhibition in non-diabetic nephropathies with non-nephrotic proteinuria. Lancet. 1999;354(9176):359–64.
44. PROGRESS Collaborative Group. Randomised trial of a perindopril-based blood-pressure-lowering regimen among 6,105 individuals with previous stroke or transient ischaemic attack. Lancet. 2001;358(9287):1033–41.
45. Bakris GL, Weir MR. Angiotensin-converting enzyme inhibitor-associated elevations in serum creatinine: is this a cause for concern? Arch Intern Med. 2000;160(5):685–93.
46. Brown MJ et al. Better blood pressure control: how to combine drugs. J Hum Hypertens. 2003;17(2):81–6.

# Chapter 5
# Congestive Heart Failure

## Definition and Epidemiology

Congestive heart failure (CHF) can be defined as the inability of the heart to provide an adequate cardiac output without invoking maladaptive compensatory mechanisms. CHF affects more than 5.7 million patients in the US – 2.5% of the adult population [1]. Five million and fifty thousand patients develop heart failure for the first time every year, and CHF results in 280,000 cardiovascular deaths and 1,100,000 hospital admissions per year in the US [1]. CHF is now the most common reason for hospitalization in the elderly, and annual costs are estimated at more than $39 billion [1]. The incidence of heart failure has been increasing, not only due to the aging of the population but also because improved treatment of hypertension and coronary disease is allowing patients to avoid early mortality only to develop heart failure later.

The causes of heart failure are protean, and are listed in Table 5.1. The predominant causes, however, are ischemia, hypertension, alcoholic cardiomyopathy, myocarditis, and idiopathic cardiomyopathy. Coronary artery disease is increasing, both as a primary cause and as a complicating factor.

Heart failure can be broken down into several different classifications: acute vs. chronic, left-sided vs. right-sided, systolic vs. diastolic dysfunction. It is important for the clinician to distinguish between systolic and diastolic dysfunction, as both the diagnostic workup and therapeutic sequence differ. Although CHF results most commonly from decreased systolic performance, diastolic dysfunction, defined clinically as cardiogenic pulmonary congestion in the presence of normal systolic performance, is becoming more common as a cause of CHF, particularly in the elderly. The estimated prevalence of diastolic heart failure is 30–35% overall, and more than 50% in patients older than 70 [2].

The severity of chronic heart failure is most commonly delineated using the classification developed by the New York Heart Association (NYHA). This classification divides patients into functional classes depending on the degree of effort needed to elicit symptoms (see Table 5.2). More recently, stages in the evolution of heart failure have been proposed by an ACC/AHA task force, to emphasize its

S. Hollenberg and S. Heitner, *Cardiology in Family Practice: A Practical Guide*, 91
Current Clinical Practice 1, DOI 10.1007/978-1-61779-385-1_5,
© Springer Science+Business Media, LLC 2012

**Table 5.1** Etiologies of
congestive heart failure

| |
| --- |
| Ischemic |
| Hypertensive |
| Idiopathic |
| Valvular |
| Peripartum |
| Familial |
| Toxic |
|   Alcoholic |
|   Radiation |
|   Drug-related (anthracyclines) |
|   Heavy metals (cobalt, lead, arsenic) |
| Metabolic/nutritional |
| Systemic diseases |
|   Hypothyroidism |
|   Connective tissue disease |
|   Diabetes |
|   Sarcoidosis |
| Infiltrative |
|   Amyloidosis |
|   Hemochromatosis |
| Tachycardia-induced |
| Autoimmune |

**Table 5.2** New York Heart Association functional classification of heart failure

| |
| --- |
| Class I: Symptoms of heart failure only at levels that would limit normal individuals |
| Class II: Symptoms of heart failure with ordinary exertion |
| Class III: Symptoms of heart failure on less than ordinary exertion |
| Class IV: Symptoms of heart failure at rest |

progressive nature and to focus on preventive measures and early intervention (see Table 5.3). These stages have been linked to therapeutic approaches (see Fig. 5.1).

**Table 5.3** Stages of heart failure

| |
| --- |
| Stage A: High risk for heart failure, without structural disease or symptoms |
| Stage B: Heart disease with asymptomatic left ventricular dysfunction |
| Stage C: Prior or current symptoms of heart failure |
| Stage D: Advanced heart disease and severely symptomatic or refractory heart failure |

## Pathophysiology

Heart failure is a syndrome caused not only by the low cardiac output resulting from compromised systolic performance, but also by the effects of compensatory mechanisms. Myocardial damage from any cause can produce myocardial failure.

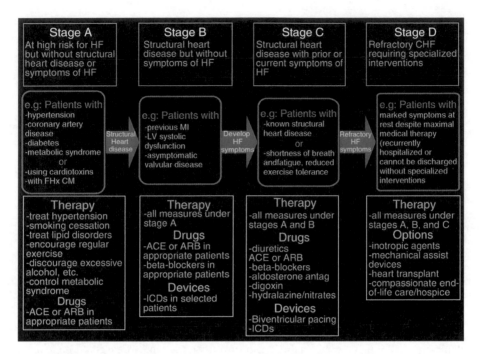

**Fig. 5.1** Stages in the evolution of heart failure and recommended therapy by stage. *HF* heart failure; *CHF* congestive heart failure; *FHx CM* family history of cardiomyopathy; *MI* myocardial infarction; *LV* left ventricular; *ACE* angiotensin-converting enzyme; *ARB* angiotensin receptor blocker; *ICD* implantable cardiac defibrillator; *CRT* cardiac resynchronization therapy

To compensate for the reduced cardiac output of a failing heart, an elevation in ventricular filling pressure occurs in an attempt to maintain output via the Frank–Starling law. These elevated diastolic filling pressures can compromise subendocardial blood flow and cause or worsen ischemia. With continued low cardiac output, additional compensatory mechanisms come into play, including sympathetic nervous system stimulation, activation of the renin-angiotensin system, and vasopressin secretion. All of these mechanisms lead to sodium and water retention and venoconstriction, increasing both preload and afterload. These increases in preload and afterload, although initially compensatory, can exacerbate heart failure, because elevated preload increases pulmonary congestion, and elevated afterload impedes cardiac output.

Recent attention has focused on cardiac remodeling, the process by which ventricular size, shape, and function are regulated by mechanical, neurohormonal, and genetic factors, as a pathophysiologic mechanism in heart failure. Remodeling may be physiological and adaptive during normal growth, but excessive remodeling after myocardial infarction, cardiomyopathy, hypertension, or valvular heart disease can be maladaptive [3]. Early local remodeling after myocardial infarction may expand the infarct zone, but late remodeling, which likely involves neurohormonal mechanisms initiated by hemodynamic stress, involves the left ventricle globally and is associated with dilation that increases over time, distortion of ventricular shape, and hypertrophy of the walls. Failure to normalize increased wall stresses results in progressive dilatation and deterioration in contractile function. Similar processes are operative in other sorts of cardiomyopathy as well. Ventricular remodeling can be considered a primary target for treatment and a reliable surrogate for long-term outcomes [3].

## Diagnosis

The symptoms and signs of CHF relate both to low cardiac output and elevated ventricular filling pressures. Low output produces the symptoms of weakness and fatigue and an ashen appearance, sometimes with mottling. Increased left-sided filling pressures result in symptoms of pulmonary congestion such as dyspnea, cough, orthopnea, and paroxysmal nocturnal dyspnea as well as signs that may include tachycardia, pulmonary rales, a diffuse, enlarged and laterally displaced point of maximal impulse, an S3 and S4 gallop, and a murmur of mitral regurgitation. Elevated right-sided preload can lead to symptoms such as anorexia, nausea, and abdominal pain along with signs of systemic congestion such as jugular venous distension, a right-sided S3 gallop, a murmur of tricuspid regurgitation, hepato-megaly, ascites, and peripheral edema.

The presentation of acute heart failure and pulmonary edema can be dramatic, with sudden onset of shortness of breath and tachypnea with use of accessory mus-cles. Crackles and often wheezing can be heard throughout the lung fields, at times obscuring some of the cardiac auscultatory findings. Hypotension and evidence of peripheral vasoconstriction and hypoperfusion may be present if cardiac output is decreased. The differential diagnosis of cardiac pulmonary edema includes other causes of acute dyspnea such as pulmonary embolism, pneumothorax, and bronchial asthma and causes of noncardiac pulmonary edema such as aspiration, infection, toxins, or trauma.

Initial evaluation of the patient with pulmonary edema should include an electro-cardiogram and chest X-ray. The electrocardiogram may show evidence of myocar-dial ischemia and can also detect arrhythmias; conduction abnormalities such as AV block and bundle branch block may be diagnosed. Q waves indicative of previous infarction or criteria diagnostic of ventricular hypertrophy may provide clues about the substrate for heart failure; atrial enlargement speaks to chronicity of elevated filling pressures. The chest X-ray can demonstrate pulmonary vascular redistribu-tion, with or without bilateral hazy pulmonary infiltrates, classically perihilar, as well as cardiomegaly. Pleural effusions may be identified but are neither sensitive nor specific.

Laboratory evaluation should include baseline serum electrolytes and creatinine, blood glucose to detect underlying diabetes, liver function tests, which may indi-cate hepatic congestion, and a complete blood count, since anemia can exacerbate preexisting CHF.

Recently, measurement of plasma B-type natriuretic peptide has been introduced into the diagnostic algorithm for CHF. BNP is produced by ventricular myocytes in response to increased wall stress (i.e., increased filling pressures and stretch). Plasma BNP levels are increased in heart failure and plasma concentration of BNP has been shown to correlate with NYHA functional class. Measurement of BNP has been used to distinguish between heart failure and pulmonary causes of dyspnea. In Breathing Not Properly (BNP) study, plasma BNP was measured with a rapid assay in 1,586 patients presenting to the emergency room with a chief complaint of dyspnea; 47% were diagnosed with CHF, 49% no CHF, and 5% were felt to have non-cardiac dyspnea in the setting of LV dysfunction [4]. Plasma BNP greater than 400 pg/mL accurately predicted CHF, while levels less than 100 pg/mL indicated noncardiac dyspnea; values between 100 and 400 pg/mL were less useful [4]. Such intermediate values may be due to CHF but may also represent preexisting LV dysfunction or right-sided failure. Addition of echocardiography in the acute setting may be especially valuable in patients with intermediate BNP levels [5].

Echocardiography can provide important information about cardiac size and function and should be performed in all patients with new onset heart failure. Echocardiography is simple, safe, and can help to provide data regarding cardiac chamber size, both left and right ventricular function, valvular structure and motion, atrial size, and the anatomy of the pericardial space. Regional wall motion abnormalities are suggestive of coronary heart disease, but are less helpful when none of the walls move normally, as conduction abnormalities can produce regional variation. Fibrotic and thinned akinetic areas, however, do indicate previous infarction. Doppler echocardiography can be used to evaluate the severity of mitral and tricuspid regurgitation, and the tricuspid regurgitation velocity can be used to estimate pulmonary artery pressure. In addition, Doppler echocardiography is increasingly used in the diagnosis of diastolic dysfunction.

Cardiovascular myocardial resonance imaging (MRI) is a rapidly evolving technology that is being used increasingly to evaluate patients with heart failure. MRI can provide accurate assessment of myocardial anatomy, regional and global function, and viability [6]. MRI may provide clues about the etiology of heart failure. With gadolinium contrast administration, early enhancement can be used to evaluate perfusion and acute tissue edema [6]. In ischemic cardiomyopathy, late hyperenhancement may reveal evidence of transmural or subendocardial infarction. In cases of nonischemic cardiomyopathy, MRI may suggest diagnoses by revealing infiltration or late gadolinium enhancement in mid-wall or epicardial regions [6].

Patients presenting with heart failure should be assessed for the presence of coronary heart disease, and thus stress testing should be considered. Either nuclear or echocardiographic imaging is usually added to increase sensitivity, although both present interpretive pitfalls in patients with severe global ventricular dysfunction. Many patients may be better served by proceeding directly to diagnostic cardiac catheterization. Even in the presence of known coronary atherosclerosis, however, stress testing may be useful to identify viable myocardium if revascularization is under consideration. In patients with severe heart failure, measurement of maximal oxygen uptake with exercise can provide an extremely useful prognostic measure [7].

Cardiac catheterization represents the gold standard for exclusion of significant coronary disease, and should be considered in most patients with new onset heart failure, even those without anginal symptoms, unless comorbid conditions render the risk prohibitive or would preclude any invasive therapy. In addition to coronary angiography, measurements of cardiac output and filling pressures can be useful both prognostically and therapeutically. Endomyocardial biopsy can be performed in selected cases if an unusual cause of myocarditis is suspected.

# Therapy

## *Treatment Goals*

The goals of CHF therapy are to control symptoms, improve exercise tolerance, prolong life, and where possible, to correct the underlying cause. Different therapies can have disparate effects on these goals.

The therapeutic agents can be viewed in the light of the pathophysiologic mechanisms of CHF development. Traditionally, these have been considered in hemodynamic terms. Fluid restriction, diuretics, and venodilators decrease cardiac preload. Angiotensin-converting enzyme (ACE) inhibitors, angiotensin receptor blockers (ARBs), and aldosterone antagonists counteract activation of the renin-angiotensin-aldosterone system and reduce afterload as well. Arterial dilators can also reduce afterload. Inotropic agents can improve cardiac pump function and increase output. More recently, effects of therapy on counterproductive neurohormonal activation have received attention. Beta blockers can counteract sympathetic activation and are being used more commonly in heart failure management. The most current approaches, however, take into account the effects of different therapies on ventricular remodeling. Therapies that have been shown to have a beneficial effect on remodeling, such as ACE inhibitors, ARBs, aldosterone antagonists, and beta blockers, reduce mortality and are effective across the whole spectrum of heart failure severity. Mechanical approaches to remodeling, most notably cardiac resynchronization therapy (CRT), are also effective.

## *General Measures*

The first order of business in the therapy of new or decompensated CHF is to address the precipitating causes, the most prominent of which are listed in Table 5.4. Bypass surgery or percutaneous intervention for cardiac ischemia can improve both symptoms and ventricular performance. Registry data consistently support the notion that in the presence of significant amounts of ischemic yet viable myocardium, revascularization confers a survival benefit [8]. For patients with symptomatic arrhythmias, either cardioversion or rate control can produce marked improvement.

| **Table 5.4**  Precipitating causes of congestive heart failure | |
|---|---|
| | Myocardial ischemia or infarction |
| | Excess salt or fluid intake |
| | Noncompliance or inadequate drug regimen |
| | Renal failure |
| | Arrhythmias |
| | Anemia |
| | Infection |
| | Fever |
| | Thytotoxicosis |
| | Pregnancy |
| | Pulmonary embolism |

Patients with acute heart failure should be put at bed rest (which by itself can produce a diuresis), with sodium restriction to less than 2 g/day and fluid restriction in severe cases. Attention should be paid to prophylaxis for deep venous thrombosis.

## Pharmacologic Therapy

### *Diuretics*

Diuretics cause renal sodium and water loss, decreasing preload and thus pulmonary and systemic congestion. For inpatient treatment of decompensated heart failure, loop diuretics such as furosemide are usually chosen initially because of their rapid onset and are given as intravenous boluses. When used for patients who present with pulmonary edema, most of the rapid effect of furosemide is attributable to venodilation.

If there is no response to a bolus dose of a loop diuretic, the dose is titrated to achieve desired effect, usually by doubling the dose. Loop diuretics enter the glomerulus primarily by tubular secretion in the proximal tubule and so exhibit a threshold effect. Once the effective dose has been determined, the degree of diuresis is usually adjusted by changing the frequency of diuretic administration. If intermittent bolus doses of loop diuretics are ineffective or are poorly tolerated due to large fluid shifts and consequent hypotension, continuous infusion may be preferable [9]. Alternatively, another diuretic with a different mechanism of action, such as metolazone or chlorthiazide may be added.

There were little clinical trial data about dosage and route of administration of diuretics in heart failure until an NIH-sponsored study randomized 308 patients with acute decompensated heart failure to either high- or low-dose furosemide and either bolus or continuous infusion, with global symptom score (efficacy) and change in creatinine (safety) as co-primary endpoints [10]. Bolus and continuous infusion did not differ in either efficacy or safety. High-dose furosemide produced greater diuresis and freedom from dyspnea at 72 h but the change in the global symptom score did not reach statistical significance; renal function did not differ either [10].

Use of diuretics can lead to significant hypokalemia or hypomagnesemia, which can predispose the patient to arrhythmias. Careful addition of a potassium-sparing diuretic can be considered in some settings.

## Nitrates

Nitroglycerin is a powerful venodilator with mild arteriolar vasodilatory effects, as well as selective coronary vasodilatory effects [11]. In vascular smooth muscle cells, nitroglycerin is biotransformed into nitrogen oxides and mimics the effects of nitric oxide, activating intracellular soluble guanylate cyclase and thus elevating cyclic GMP levels.

Nitroglycerin relieves pulmonary congestion acutely primarily through direct venodilation – reducing left ventricular filling pressures, wall stress, and myocardial oxygen consumption – decreasing left ventricular filling pressures [11]. At higher doses, coronary artery dilation and increased collateral blood flow may improve ischemia, an effect often desirable given the high incidence of coronary artery disease in patients with CHF. In acute heart failure, intravenous nitroglycerin has been shown to decrease both right and left ventricular filling pressures, as well as systemic vascular resistance [12].

Nitrates are first-line agents for the symptomatic relief of angina pectoris and when myocardial infarction is complicated by CHF. Given the high incidence of coronary artery disease in patients with CHF, use of nitrates to reduce preload is often desirable. In severely decompensated CHF, intravenous nitroglycerin is preferred because of questionable absorption of oral and transdermal preparations and for ease of titration. Intravenous nitroglycerin should be started at 5 μg/min and increased in increments of 5 μg/min every 3–5 min as needed for symptomatic relief. Use of nitroglycerin can be limited by side effects, most prominently hypotension and headache, and by nitrate tolerance, with attenuation of its hemodynamic effects [12]. Because of the development of tolerance, nitroglycerin doses may need to be increased dramatically. In a report of a single center experience with intravenous nitroglycerin as part of the Vasodilation in the Management of Acute Congestive (VMAC) heart failure trial, nitroglycerin doses had to be increased from a mean of 40–160 μg/min to maintain a reduction in wedge pressure at 12 h, and even then, the effect was attenuated at 24 h [13]. This finding underscores the need for close monitoring and frequent dose titration in patients with acute heart failure.

Long-term therapy with oral nitrates alone does not impact ventricular remodeling and thus, in the absence of ongoing ischemia, is not usually a first-line choice. When combined with hydralazine, however, salutary effects on outcome have been demonstrated, first in the V-HeFT trial [14], and more recently in the A-HeFT trial [15]. These trials are described below in the section on hydralazine.

## Angiotensin-Converting Enzyme Inhibitors

ACE inhibitors inhibit conversion of angiotensin I to angiotensin II and also inhibit breakdown of bradykinin. Both of these actions produce vasodilation, the latter through bradykinin-induced nitric oxide production, but the increased inhibition of ventricular remodeling seen with ACE inhibitors compared to other vasodilators speaks to the potential for involvement of other mechanisms. Local renin-angiotensin systems, both intracardiac and intravascular, contribute to myocardial hypertrophy and remodeling, and their inhibition by ACE inhibitors may explain part of their beneficial effects [16].

ACE inhibitors improve hemodynamics, functional capacity, and survival in patients across the spectrum of severity of chronic CHF and also after myocardial infarction. The CONSENSUS study group compared enalapril to placebo in 253 patients with advanced heart failure (NYHA class III or IV) and showed a 40% reduction in 6-month mortality; this benefit was sustained, with a risk reduction averaged over the 10 year duration of the trial of 30% [17]. The SOLVD treatment trial compared enalapril to placebo in 2,569 patients with symptomatic heart failure (NYHA class II–III) and showed a 16% mortality reduction [18]. Moreover, ACE inhibitors also prevented the development of CHF in patients with asymptomatic left ventricular dysfunction in the SOLVD prevention trial [19].

ACE inhibitors also improve the outcome in patients with asymptomatic LV dysfunction or overt heart failure after an acute MI. In the SAVE trial, 2,231 asymptomatic patients with an ejection fraction less than 40% were randomly assigned to either captopril or placebo. Captopril decreased mortality by 19% at 42 months, and also decreased hospitalization for heart failure, and, interestingly, recurrent MI [20]. The latter effect may have been due to improvement in endothelial function. The AIRE trial compared ramipril to placebo in 2,006 patients with clinical heart failure and showed a 27% reduction in mortality at 15 months [21]. The survival benefit was maintained long term in both trials.

Patients should be started on low doses and titrated upward to the range demonstrated beneficial in clinical trials (captopril 50 mg thrice daily, enalapril 20 mg twice daily, or lisinopril 40 mg once daily). Side effects of ACE inhibitors include cough, renal failure (usually occurs in the setting of renal artery stenosis), hyperkalemia, and angioedema.

## Angiotensin Receptor Blockers

An alternative approach to inhibiting the effects of angiotensin II is use of agents that block the angiotensin II receptor (ARBs). Since these agents do not increase bradykinin, the incidence of some side effects, such as cough and angioedema, is greatly reduced. The hemodynamic effects of ARBs are similar to those of ACE inhibitors, and trials comparing ACE inhibitors to ARBs in patients with heart failure have shown similar mortality reductions [22–26].

The recent recognition that angiotensin II is produced by pathways other than ACE has provided a rationale for using ACE inhibitors and ARBs in combination. This approach was tested in the Valsartan in Heart Failure (Val-HeFT) trial, in which valsartan or placebo was added to usual therapy in patients with heart failure [22]. The primary endpoint of overall mortality was unchanged, although the combined endpoint of mortality and hospital admission for CHF was reduced with valsartan [22]. In the VALIANT trial, which compared valsartan, captopril, and the combination of the two in patients with acute MI and CHF, mortality did not differ among the three groups [23]. The incidence of side effects was similar between valsartan and captopril, but was increased when both were given [23]. Similar results were seen in the more recent and much larger ONTARGET trial, which randomized 25,557 patients with vascular disease or diabetes but without heart failure, to the ACE inhibitor ramipril, the ARB telmisartan, or the combination of the two drugs [27]. There was no difference in the primary outcome, the combination of death, MI, stroke, or heart failure hospitalization, despite a reduction in blood pressure in the combination group [27]. Telmisartan led to less cough and angioedema, but more symptomatic hypotension, the combination of telmisartan with ramipril increased side effects compared to monotherapy [27].

Thus, the available data indicate that ARBs are likely as effective, but not more effective than ACE inhibitors, with a different side effect profile and substantially increased cost. The ACC/AHA guidelines recommend that an ARB should be used for treating heart failure in patients who cannot tolerate an ACE inhibitor [7]. There is no compelling data that addition of ARBs to ACE inhibitors improves outcomes, but this strategy might be employed in selected patients with heart failure in whom blood pressure proves difficult to control with other agents.

## Aldosterone Antagonists

Although aldosterone is predominantly known for its role in regulation of renal sodium and potassium excretion, its neurohumoral effects are gaining increasing recognition. In addition to its effects on fluid retention, aldosterone inhibition inhibits cardiac fibrosis and ventricular remodeling as well.

The RALES trial randomized 1,653 patients with class III and IV heart failure to spironolactone or placebo, and found a reduction in 24-month mortality from 46 to 35% (RR 30%, $p < 0.001$) [28]. Hyperkalemia was uncommon, and the main side effect was gynecomastia. The EPHESUS trial randomized 6,632 patients with left ventricular dysfunction after MI (class I and II heart failure) to the aldosterone antagonist eplerenone or placebo, and found a 15% reduction in mortality (RR 0.85, CI 0.75–0.96, $p < 0.01$) [29]. In this trial, hyperkalemia was noted in 5.5% of the eplerenone group compared to 3.9% of the placebo group ($p < 0.01$), but interestingly, hypokalemia was reduced, from 13.1 to 8.4% [29]. Recently, the EMPHASIS trial randomized 2,737 patients with class II heart failure and ejection fraction <35% to eplerenone or placebo; the trial was stopped early because of a significant 24%

reduction in both death (3% absolute reduction) and the combination of mortality and heart failure hospitalization (7.6% absolute reduction) in the eplerenone group [30]. Hyperkalemia was increased with eplerenone in this trial as well [30].

It should be noted that the doses of aldosterone antagonists used in these heart failure trials were well below those used for diuresis. Nonetheless, careful attention to serum potassium levels is warranted when using these agents for any indication, and they should not be used in patients with substantial renal insufficiency (estimated glomerular filtration rate <30 mL/min).

## Beta Blockers

Symptomatic heart failure results in activation of neurohumoral mechanisms, including the sympathetic nervous system, that initially support the performance of the failing heart. Long-term activation of the sympathetic nervous system, however, exerts deleterious effects. Circulating catecholamine levels correlate with survival in these patients [31]. Sympathetic activation can increase ventricular volumes and pressure by causing peripheral vasoconstriction and by impairing sodium excretion by the kidneys and can also provoke arrhythmias. Chronic stimulation of beta receptors reduces the responsiveness to beta adrenergic agonists due to downregulation and desensitization of the beta receptor and its coupled signaling pathways, and beta blockade can upregulate adrenergic receptor density, restoring inotropic and chronotropic responsiveness [7]. Catecholamines induce oxidative stress in cardiac myocytes, potentially leading to programmed cell death, a process counteracted by beta blockers [32]. Beta blockers also reduce the circulating level of vasoconstrictors and mitigate their effects, decreasing afterload. Perhaps most importantly, catecholamines promote deleterious ventricular remodeling, and beta blockers can decrease left ventricular end-systolic and end-diastolic volume [7]. Thus, although, perhaps counterintuitive on hemodynamic grounds, there is now compelling evidence that beta blockers are beneficial not only for patients with acute myocardial infarction complicated by heart failure but also with chronic heart failure from all causes [7].

Beta blockers have now been evaluated in more than 10,000 patients with heart failure and systolic dysfunction. This collective experience indicates that long-term treatment with beta blockers can relieve symptoms, improve ventricular performance, and reduce both mortality and the need for hospitalization. Three different agents have been shown to decrease mortality in patients with class II and III heart failure: metoprolol XL [33], bisoprolol [34], and carvedilol [35]. Additional studies with carvedilol indicate that the benefits extend to patients with class IV heart failure [36]. These benefits of beta blockers are seen in patients with or without coronary artery disease and in patients with or without diabetes, and are also observed in patients already taking ACE inhibitors.

Initiation of beta blockers, however, can be problematic during the acute phase of heart failure, as they can depress contractility. When given for heart failure indications, beta blockers should be introduced when the patient is in a well compensated and euvolemic state, starting with low doses. Patients who experience an exacerbation of heart failure while on maintenance beta blocker therapy, particularly at a higher dose, present a previously rare dilemma that is becoming more common. No controlled observations are available to guide therapy, so current practice remains largely at the discretion of individual clinicians. Discontinuing beta blockers, or decreasing their dose, may expose myocardial beta receptors to endogenous catecholamines, and may result in a brief increase in contractility. On the other hand, slow titration of beta blockers will need to begin anew after resolution of acute CHF. It is usually best to attempt to resolve acute episodes of heart failure by diuresis and adjustment of other medications while holding beta blocker doses constant. If that approach is unsuccessful, the next step is to halve the dose. If heart failure persists, and particularly if inotropic therapy is required, then beta blockers may need to be discontinued, but every attempt should be made to restart them once the acute exacerbation of CHF has resolved.

## Hydralazine

Hydralazine reduces afterload by directly relaxing smooth muscle. Its effects are almost exclusively confined to the arterial bed. In normal subjects, the hypotensive actions of hydralazine provoke a marked reflex tachycardia, but this response is often blunted in subjects with heart failure.

Hydralazine is effective in increasing cardiac output in heart failure. Hydralazine in combination with oral nitrates was the first therapy shown to improve mortality in CHF when given, reducing mortality in patients with class III and IV heart failure in the V-HeFT trial [14]. Enalapril was shown to be superior to this combination [37]. In addition, oral hydralazine must be given thrice a day, and prolonged administration is attended by the development of a lupus-like syndrome in up to 20% of patients, and so hydralazine has usually been reserved for ACE-intolerant patients.

Recently, the A-HeFT trial tested a fixed dose of both isosorbide dinitrate and hydralazine in blacks with class III and IV heart failure, a subgroup previously noted to have a favorable response to this therapy and that may not respond as well to ACE inhibition [15]. When added to ACE inhibitors and beta blockers, the combination of hydralazine and nitrates improved mortality, heart failure hospitalization, and quality of life [15].

## Nesiritide

Nesiritide is a recombinant form of human B-type natriuretic peptide (BNP). BNP assays have been used in the diagnosis of heart failure as described above, but when infused intravenously, nesiritide is a vasodilator that also has a natriuretic effect. In patients with heart failure, intravenous nesiritide has been shown to increase stroke volume and cardiac output and to decrease right atrial and pulmonary capillary wedge pressure. In the VMAC trial, 489 patients, including 246 who underwent pulmonary artery catheterization, were randomly assigned to nesiritide, intravenous nitroglycerin, or placebo for 3 h, followed by nesiritide or intravenous nitroglycerin for 24 h [38]. Nesiritide decreased the mean pulmonary capillary wedge pressure PCWP significantly more than either intravenous nitroglycerin or placebo at 3 h (5.8 vs. 3.8 and 2.0 mmHg) and significantly more than nitroglycerin at 24 h (8.2 vs. 6.3 mmHg). Symptoms of dyspnea were significantly decreased compared with placebo, but compared to intravenous nitroglycerin [38].

Questions about the effect of nesiritide on renal function and mortality led to the performance of ASCEND-HF, a 7,007 patient clinical trial comparing nesiritide to placebo with combined 30-day mortality and CHF hospitalization and also dyspnea relief as efficacy endpoints and increase in creatinine as a safety endpoint in patients with decompensated heart failure [39]. There was no difference in death or hospitalization. Dyspnea score was improved significantly (in 44.5 vs. 42.1% at 6 h and 68.2 vs. 66.1% at 24 h), but these differences were small. Nesiritide neither improved nor worsened renal function. The incidence of symptomatic hypotension was greater with nesiritide [39]. Nesiritide remains an alternative for patients not responding to other therapies, but there is no compelling reason to use it as first-line therapy.

## Digoxin

Digitalis, which has been used to treat heart failure for more than 200 years, works by inhibiting Na-K-dependent ATPase activity, causing intracellular sodium accumulation and increasing intracellular calcium via the sodium–calcium exchange system. Digoxin improves myocardial contractility and increases cardiac output, but its inotropic effects are mild in comparison to catecholamines. Digoxin has been shown to improve symptoms in patients with heart failure. The effect of digoxin on survival was definitively addressed in the Digoxin Investigators' Group (DIG) trial, a study of 6,800 patients with symptomatic CHF and systolic dysfunction [40]. There was no difference in survival between the digoxin and placebo groups, but digoxin did decrease hospitalization for heart failure significantly [40]. Thus, apart from its use as an antiarrhythmic agent, digoxin is recommended in patients with systolic dysfunction, who remain symptomatic despite therapy with diuretics, ACE inhibitors, and beta blockers.

## Inotropic Agents

In severe decompensated heart failure, inotropic support may be initiated. Dobutamine is a selective $\beta_1$-adrenergic receptor agonist that can improve myocardial contractility and increase cardiac output. Dobutamine is the initial inotropic agent of choice in patients with decompensated acute heart failure and systolic blood pressure >90 mmHg. Dobutamine has a rapid onset of action and a plasma half-life of 2–3 min; infusion is usually initiated at 5 μg/kg/min and then titrated. Tolerance to the effect of dobutamine may develop after 48–72 h, possibly due to downregulation of adrenergic receptors. Dobutamine has the potential to exacerbate hypotension in some patients, and can precipitate tachyarrhythmias.

Milrinone is a phosphodiesterase inhibitor which increases cardiac contractility and also mediates vasodilation by increasing intracellular cyclic AMP. Because milrinone does not stimulate adrenergic receptors directly, it may be effective when added to catecholamines or when β-adrenergic receptors have been downregulated. Compared to catecholamines, phosphodiesterase inhibitors have fewer chronotropic and arrhythmogenic effects, but more of a propensity to produce hypotension. Milrinone was examined in a prospective manner in the OPTIME-CHF trial in order to determine whether its use could reduce hospitalization time following an acute heart failure exacerbation [41]. No benefit was found with milrinone compared to digoxin, and patients with ischemic cardiomyopathy actually had worse outcomes [42]. In OPTIME-CHF, however, patients whom the investigators felt "needed" acute inotropic support were excluded, thereby biasing the enrollment toward a less severely afflicted cohort.

Since sympathetic overstimulation is one of the causes of left ventricular remodeling with increased dimensions and decreased ejection fraction, long-term catecholamine administration might be supposed to have negative consequences, and, in fact, have been associated with increased mortality in heart failure [43]. Nonetheless, some patients with acute decompensation may benefit from hemodynamic support with dobutamine or milrinone. Inotropic infusions need to be titrated carefully in patients with ischemic heart disease to maximize coronary perfusion pressure with the least possible increase in myocardial oxygen demand. Invasive hemodynamic monitoring can be extremely useful to allow for optimization of therapy in these unstable patients, because clinical estimates of filling pressure can be unreliable, and because changes in myocardial performance and compliance and therapeutic interventions can change cardiac output and filling pressures precipitously. Optimization of filling pressures and serial measurements of cardiac output (and other parameters, such as mixed venous oxygen saturation) allow for titration of inotropes and vasopressors to the minimum dosage required to achieve the chosen therapeutic goals, thus minimizing the increases in myocardial oxygen demand and arrhythmogenic potential.

## Arrhythmias

Arrhythmias are common in patients with heart failure. Nonsustained ventricular tachycardia may occur in as many as 50% of patients, and complex ventricular depolarizations in as many as 80%. Forty to fifty percent of deaths are sudden, and many of these deaths are attributable to arrhythmias. The mortality benefits of some of the standard therapies for heart failure, particularly beta blockers, may be attributable in part to antiarrhythmic properties. Specific antiarrhythmic agents, however, have not proven very effective for the prevention of sudden death in patients with heart failure [44], and so attention is focused on identifying patients who would benefit from implantation of an implantable cardiac defibrillator (ICD).

Implantation of ICDs as secondary prevention in survivors of sudden cardiac death or patients with hemodynamically significant sustained ventricular tachycardias has been well demonstrated to improve survival in randomized clinical trials [44–47]. As secondary prevention, the AVID Study showed that patients resuscitated from ventricular fibrillation or with hemodynamically significant VT with EF ≤40% had improved survival with ICD compared to antiarrhythmic therapy (amiodarone in more than 80%) [44].

ICDs are effective as primary prevention in selected heart failure patients as well. The MADIT-I and MUSST trials showed a mortality benefit with ICD in patients with left ventricular dysfunction (EF <35–40%) and nonsustained VT in whom sustained VT was inducible at electrophysiologic study [46, 48]. The MADIT-II trial showed a mortality benefit with ICD in a trial which the entry criterion was simply an ejection fraction less than 30% [47]. Most of the patients in these trials had ischemic cardiomyopathy. The SCD-HeFT trial compared ICD implantation to amiodarone in patients with heart failure due to either an ischemic or nonischemic cardiomyopathy (EF <35%), and found a mortality benefit with ICD in both groups [45].

## Cardiac Resynchronization

Left bundle branch block or other conduction system abnormalities can cause dyssynchronous ventricular contraction. Such dyssynchrony causes abnormal septal motion, decreasing contractile performance and myocardial efficiency, reduces diastolic filling times, and can increase the duration and degree of mitral regurgitation. The goal of CRT is to pace the left and right ventricles to restore physiologic atrioventricular timing and contraction synchrony. This is accomplished by placing standard leads in the right atrium and right ventricle and also placing a special lead through the coronary sinus to enable pacing of the lateral aspect of the left ventricle.

CRT, by optimizing the coordination of contraction, improves LV contractile function, stroke volume, and cardiac output. This improved performance is associated with either no increase or a decrease in myocardial oxygen consumption, thus increasing myocardial efficiency. Most importantly, biventricular pacing decreases left ventricular diastolic and systolic dimension, mitral regurgitation, and LV mass, all signs of reverse remodeling [49]. Cardiac resynchronization also improves exercise capacity, functional class, and quality of life [49].

CRT also improves hard outcomes. The COMPANION trial compared optimal medical therapy to CRT with and without an ICD in 1,520 patients with NYHA class III or IV heart failure, an LVEF <35% and prolonged QRS duration (>120 ms) [50]. The primary endpoint, a combination of all-cause mortality and hospitalization, was reduced in both the CRT alone and the CRT plus ICD arm compared to medical therapy [50]. In the recently CARE-HF trial, cardiac resynchronization reduced the interventricular mechanical delay, which randomized patients with class III or IV CHF to resynchronization (without an ICD) or medical therapy, negative remodeling was observed, symptoms and quality of life improved, and reduced both death and, most importantly, the combined end point of death and hospitalization was reduced with CRT [51].

Recently, two studies, MADIT-CRT [52] and RAFT [53] have examined the effects of CRT on patients with less severe (NYHA Class II and III) heart failure and prolonged QRS duration. Both trials showed significant reductions in their primary end points, a combination of death and hospitalization for heart failure, and RAFT showed a reduction in all-cause mortality, a prespecified secondary outcome [52, 53]. Reverse remodeling was seen in both studies [52, 53]. Taken together, the data suggest that in appropriate candidates with evidence of ventricular dyssynchrony, CRT can prevent or reverse left ventricular remodeling in CHF, and that this reduction improves both symptoms and mortality.

## *Overview*

The goals of heart failure therapy are to reduce symptoms, improve exercise tolerance, and increase survival. While these are all worthy goals, thus far only therapies that impact ventricular remodeling have been shown to influence mortality (see Table 5.5). Therapies that either prevent or reverse remodeling also tend to be effective across the spectrum of heart failure therapy. Thus, for long-term therapy, the aim is to put patients on the therapies that have been demonstrated in clinical trials to improve mortality, and to titrate the doses of those therapies to the levels achieved in the trials.

**Table 5.5**  Remodeling and survival by drug class

| Established therapy | Remodeling effects | Survival effects |
|---|---|---|
| ACE-I | Benefit | Benefit |
| ARB | Benefit | Benefit |
| Aldosterone antagonists | Benefit | Benefit |
| β-blockers | Benefit | Benefit |
| Diuretics | No benefit | No benefit |
| Digoxin | No benefit | No benefit |
| Resynchronization (CRT) | Benefit | Benefit |
| *Other therapies* | | |
| Endothelin antagonists | No benefit | No benefit |
| TNF-α | No benefit | No benefit |
| Inotropes | Adverse | Adverse |

*ACE* angiotensin converting enzyme; *ARB* angiotensin receptor blocker; *TNF* tumor necrosis factor; *CRT* cardiac resynchronization therapy

# Diastolic Heart Failure

## Definition

There is growing recognition that a sizable number of patients with heart failure do not have a significant abnormality of systolic performance. Diastolic heart failure is a clinical syndrome characterized by the signs and symptoms of heart failure and a preserved ejection fraction.

Virtually all patients with diastolic heart failure have a measurable abnormality in ventricular diastolic performance [2]. Nonetheless, the term "diastolic dysfunction" has the potential to cause confusion. Strictly speaking, unequivocal documentation of abnormal diastolic function would require demonstration that the ventricular end-diastolic pressure volume curve is shifted upward, a task that requires simultaneous assessment of both pressure and volume across a wide range of values. What is more commonly present is evidence of elevated end-diastolic pressures or increased diastolic stiffness, a situation that may result from either a shifted compliance curve or from increased LV end-diastolic volume. Since the compensatory response to significant systolic dysfunction usually entails increased end-diastolic volume, it follows that virtually all patients with systolic dysfunction have diastolic dysfunction as well. Diastolic heart failure denotes patients with diastolic dysfunction in the absence of significant systolic dysfunction. Whether documentation of diastolic dysfunction is strictly necessary remains a bit controversial [2].

## Epidemiology

Diastolic heart failure is estimated to account for up to a third of cases of CHF, with the proportion increasing to almost 50% in the elderly. Thus, diastolic heart failure is becoming more common as the population ages.

The most common causes of diastolic heart failure are hypertension and ischemic heart disease, although other less common etiologies include hypertrophic and restrictive cardiomyopathies and some valvular abnormalities, most prominently aortic stenosis.

Although the prognosis is less ominous for patients with diastolic than systolic heart failure (annual mortality 5–8% compared to 10–15%), mortality exceeds that of age-matched controls [2]. Morbidity is high as well, with similar symptoms and readmission rates (approaching 50% at 1 year) compared to systolic heart failure [2].

## Etiology and Diagnosis

Diastolic function has a number of subtleties, and its analysis can become quite complex. Nonetheless, early diastole is the period of ventricular relaxation, and ventricular filling is most important later on. Ventricular relaxation has both active and passive components. The active component is dependent on calcium removal from the myofilaments and cytoplasm, and is energy dependent. Thus, active relaxation can be impaired by myocardial ischemia. The passive component of relaxation consists of elastic recoil of structural proteins compressed during systole. Chamber filling is reflected in the diastolic pressure-volume relation [54].

There are a variety of measures, both invasive and noninvasive, for the assessment of diastolic function. Each measurement indexes slightly different features, and none by itself embodies all of the relevant information. By taking several measures together, however, the picture becomes clearer.

Echocardiography is the most useful method for assessment of ventricular function in the clinical setting [55]. First, it provides a measure of systolic performance, allowing for distinction of systolic from diastolic heart failure. Doppler echocardiography of mitral inflow patterns generates measures of early (E velocity) and late (A, corresponding to atrial contraction) filling velocities. In normal heart, the E wave is greater than the A wave. As diastolic dysfunction develops, the E wave decreases (and deceleration time increases) and the A wave increases ("E–A reversal"). With severe diastolic dysfunction, left atrial pressure increases markedly and the E wave becomes much larger than the A wave (with a very short deceleration time), the "restrictive pattern." In between the first and last stages of diastolic dysfunction, there is a pattern known as "pseudonormalization," in which the E and A waves appear normal, but left atrial pressure is increased. Thus, relying only on these patterns and E and A velocities has the potential to generate some confusion. A number of newer and more specific echocardiographic measures are coming into clinical use, including pulmonary and hepatic vein velocities. The most promising is Tissue Doppler imaging of the mitral annulus, which moves away from the apex with ventricular filling [55]. The ratio of mitral inflow velocity to mitral annular velocity (E/E') increases with higher filling pressures; a value greater than 15 is specific for a pulmonary artery occlusion pressure greater than 20 mmHg [55].

## Management

The initial step in treating patients with diastolic heart failure is to reduce pulmonary congestion by decreasing LV volume. Maintaining synchronous atrial contraction is an important adjunct. Treatment of the underlying disease process is of clear importance as well. Blood pressure control should be optimized in hypertensive patients. If ischemia is the inciting cause, then appropriate diagnostic and therapeutic measures should be pursued.

There have been few randomized trials in patients with diastolic heart failure. The CHARM-Preserved trial randomized 3,023 patients with CHF and ejection fraction >40% to the ARB candesartan or placebo [56]. The primary outcome, cardiovascular death, or hospitalization for CHF, did not differ between groups (22 vs. 24%, HR 0.89, CI 0.77–1.03, $p=0.12$), and death was equivalent, but rates of admission were lower with candesartan [56]. The I-PRESERVE trial randomized 4,128 patients with ejection fraction >45% to the ARB irbesartan or placebo, and showed no difference in mortality, hospitalization for heart failure, or quality of life [57]. Thus, although blood pressure control is an important therapeutic goal, no particular drugs have been proven effective, specifically for diastolic heart failure.

Tachycardia is poorly tolerated in patients with diastolic heart failure, particularly those with the potential for ischemia, since myocardial oxygen demand is increased and diastolic filling times are shortened. Thus, beta blockers and calcium channel blockers with negative chronotropic effects can increase exercise tolerance and provide symptomatic improvement. Stroke volumes in patients with diastolic heart failure are generally subnormal, because despite preserved ejection fraction, left ventricular cavity size is small [58]. Doses should be individualized with the goal of blunting the tachycardic response to stress and exercise without unduly decreasing resting heart rate and cardiac output.

# References

1. Lloyd-Jones D, Adams RJ, Brown TM, et al. Heart disease and stroke statistics – 2010 update: a report from the American Heart Association. Circulation. 2010;121:e46–215.
2. Zile MR, Brutsaert DL. New concepts in diastolic dysfunction and diastolic heart failure: Part I: diagnosis, prognosis, and measurements of diastolic function. Part II: causal mechanisms and treatment. Circulation. 2002;105(1387–93):503–8.
3. Sutton MG, Sharpe N. Left ventricular remodeling after myocardial infarction: pathophysiology and therapy. Circulation. 2000;101:2981–8.
4. Maisel AS, Krishnaswamy P, Nowak RM, et al. Rapid measurement of B-type natriuretic peptide in the emergency diagnosis of heart failure. N Engl J Med. 2002;347:161–7.
5. Logeart D, Saudubray C, Beyne P, et al. Comparative value of Doppler echocardiography and B-type natriuretic peptide assay in the etiologic diagnosis of acute dyspnea. J Am Coll Cardiol. 2002;40:1794–800.
6. Karamitsos TD, Francis JM, Myerson S, Selvanayagam JB, Neubauer S. The role of cardiovascular magnetic resonance imaging in heart failure. J Am Coll Cardiol. 2009;54:1407–24.
7. Hunt SA, Abraham WT, Chin MH, et al. ACC/AHA 2005 guideline update for the diagnosis and management of chronic heart failure in the adult-summary article. J Am Coll Cardiol. 2005;46:1116–43.
8. CASS Principal Investigators. A randomized trial of coronary artery bypass surgery. Survival of patients with a low ejection fraction. N Engl J Med. 1985;312:1665–71.
9. Dormans TP, van Meyel JJ, Gerlag PG, Tan Y, Russel FG, Smits P. Diuretic efficacy of high dose furosemide in severe heart failure: bolus injection versus continuous infusion. J Am Coll Cardiol. 1996;28:376–82.
10. Felker GM, Lee KL, Bull DA, et al. Diuretic strategies in patients with acute decompensated heart failure. N Engl J Med. 2011;364:797–805.
11. Cohn PF, Gorlin R. Physiologic and clinical actions of nitroglycerin. Med Clin North Am. 1974;58:407–15.
12. Elkayam U, Bitar F, Akhter MW, Khan S, Patrus S, Derakhshani M. Intravenous nitroglycerin in the treatment of decompensated heart failure: potential benefits and limitations. J Cardiovasc Pharmacol Ther. 2004;9:227–41.
13. Elkayam U, Akhter MW, Singh H, Khan S, Usman A. Comparison of effects on left ventricular filling pressure of intravenous nesiritide and high-dose nitroglycerin in patients with decompensated heart failure. Am J Cardiol. 2004;93:237–40.
14. Cohn JN, Archibald DG, Ziesche S, et al. Effect of vasodilator therapy on mortality in chronic congestive heart failure. Results of a Veterans Administration cooperative study. N Engl J Med. 1986;314:1547–52.

15. Taylor AL, Ziesche S, Yancy C, et al. Combination of isosorbide dinitrate and hydralazine in blacks with heart failure. N Engl J Med. 2004;351:2049–57.
16. Dzau VJ, Bernstein K, Celermajer D, et al. The relevance of tissue angiotensin-converting enzyme: manifestations in mechanistic and endpoint data. Am J Cardiol. 2001;88:1L–20.
17. CONSENSUS Trial Study Group. Effects of enalapril on mortality in severe congestive heart failure. Results of the Cooperative North Scandanavian Enalapril Survival Study (CONSENSUS). N Engl J Med. 1987;316:1429–35.
18. Investigators SOLVD. Effect of enalapril on survival in patients with reduced left ventricular ejection fractions and congestive heart failure. N Engl J Med. 1991;325:293–302.
19. Investigators SOLVD. Effect of enalapril on mortality and the development of heart failure in asymptomatic patients with reduced left ventricular ejection fractions. N Engl J Med. 1992; 327:685–91.
20. Pfeffer MA, Braunwald E, Moye LA, et al. Effect of captopril on mortality and morbidity in patients with left ventricular dysfunction after myocardial infarction. Results of the Survival and Ventricular Enlargement Trial. N Engl J Med. 1992;327:669–77.
21. Acute Infarction Ramipril Efficacy (AIRE) Study Investigators. Effect of ramipril on mortality and morbidity of survivors of acute myocardial infarction with clinical evidence of heart failure. Lancet. 1993;342:821–8.
22. Cohn JN, Tognoni G. A randomized trial of the angiotensin-receptor blocker valsartan in chronic heart failure. N Engl J Med. 2001;345:1667–75.
23. Pfeffer MA, McMurray JJ, Velazquez EJ, et al. Valsartan, captopril, or both in myocardial infarction complicated by heart failure, left ventricular dysfunction, or both. N Engl J Med. 2003;349:1893–906.
24. Pfeffer MA, Swedberg K, Granger CB, et al. Effects of candesartan on mortality and morbidity in patients with chronic heart failure: the CHARM-Overall programme. Lancet. 2003;362:759–66.
25. Pitt B, Poole-Wilson PA, Segal R, et al. Effect of losartan compared with captopril on mortality in patients with symptomatic heart failure: randomised trial – the Losartan Heart Failure Survival Study ELITE II. Lancet. 2000;355:1582–7.
26. McMurray JJ, Ostergren J, Swedberg K, et al. Effects of candesartan in patients with chronic heart failure and reduced left-ventricular systolic function taking angiotensin-converting-enzyme inhibitors: the CHARM-Added trial. Lancet. 2003;362:767–71.
27. Yusuf S, Teo KK, Pogue J, et al. Telmisartan, ramipril, or both in patients at high risk for vascular events. N Engl J Med. 2008;358:1547–59.
28. Pitt B, Zannad F, Remme WJ, et al. The effect of spironolactone on morbidity and mortality in patients with severe heart failure. N Engl J Med. 1999;341:709–17.
29. Pitt B, Remme W, Zannad F, et al. Eplerenone, a selective aldosterone blocker, in patients with left ventricular dysfunction after myocardial infarction. N Engl J Med. 2003;348:1309–21.
30. Zannad F, McMurray JJ, Krum H, et al. Eplerenone in patients with systolic heart failure and mild symptoms. N Engl J Med. 2011;364:11–21.
31. Cohn JN, Levine TB, Olivari MT, et al. Plasma norepinephrine as a guide to prognosis in patients with chronic congestive heart failure. N Engl J Med. 1984;311:819–23.
32. Lohse MJ, Engelhardt S, Eschenhagen T. What is the role of beta-adrenergic signaling in heart failure? Circ Res. 2003;93:896–906.
33. Metoprolol CR/XL Randomised Intervention Trial in Congestive Heart Failure Investigators. Effect of metoprolol CR/XL in chronic heart failure: Metoprolol CR/XL Randomised Intervention Trial in Congestive Heart Failure (MERIT-HF). Lancet. 1999;353:2001–7.
34. Investigators CIBIS-II. The Cardiac Insufficiency Bisoprolol Study II (CIBIS-II): a randomised trial. Lancet. 1999;353:9–13.
35. Packer M, Coats AJ, Fowler MB, et al. Effect of carvedilol on survival in severe chronic heart failure. N Engl J Med. 2001;344:1651–8.
36. Krum H, Roecker EB, Mohacsi P, et al. Effects of initiating carvedilol in patients with severe chronic heart failure: results from the COPERNICUS Study. JAMA. 2003;289:712–8.

37. Cohn JN, Johnson G, Ziesche S, et al. A comparison of enalapril with hydralazine-isosorbide dinitrate in the treatment of chronic congestive heart failure. N Engl J Med. 1991;325: 303–10.
38. Investigators VMAC. Intravenous nesiritide vs nitroglycerin for treatment of decompensated congestive heart failure: a randomized controlled trial. JAMA. 2002;287:1531–40.
39. ASCEND Trial Investigators. Acute study of clinical effectiveness of nesiritide in decompensated heart failure. in press 2011.
40. Digitalis Investigation Group. The effect of digoxin on mortality and morbidity in patients with heart failure. N Engl J Med. 1997;336:525–33.
41. Cuffe MS, Califf RM, Adams Jr KF, et al. Short-term intravenous milrinone for acute exacerbation of chronic heart failure: a randomized controlled trial. JAMA. 2002;287:1541–7.
42. Felker GM, Benza RL, Chandler AB, et al. Heart failure etiology and response to milrinone in decompensated heart failure: results from the OPTIME-CHF study. J Am Coll Cardiol. 2003;41:997–1003.
43. O'Connor CM, Gattis WA, Uretsky BF, et al. Continuous intravenous dobutamine is associated with an increased risk of death in patients with advanced heart failure: insights from the Flolan International Randomized Survival Trial (FIRST). Am Heart J. 1999;138:78–86.
44. Antiarrhythmics Versus Implantable Defibrillators (AVID) Investigators. A comparison of antiarrhythmic-drug therapy with implantable defibrillators in patients resuscitated from near-fatal ventricular arrhythmias. The Antiarrhythmics versus Implantable Defibrillators (AVID) Investigators. N Engl J Med. 1997;337:1576–83.
45. Bardy GH, Lee KL, Mark DB, et al. Amiodarone or an implantable cardioverter-defibrillator for congestive heart failure. N Engl J Med. 2005;352:225–37.
46. Buxton AE, Lee KL, Fisher JD, Josephson ME, Prystowsky EN, Hafley G. A randomized study of the prevention of sudden death in patients with coronary artery disease. Multicenter Unsustained Tachycardia Trial Investigators. N Engl J Med. 1999;341:1882–90.
47. Moss AJ, Zareba W, Hall WJ, et al. Prophylactic implantation of a defibrillator in patients with myocardial infarction and reduced ejection fraction. N Engl J Med. 2002;346:877–83.
48. Moss AJ, Hall WJ, Cannom DS, et al. Improved survival with an implanted defibrillator in patients with coronary disease at high risk for ventricular arrhythmia. N Engl J Med. 1996; 335:1933–40.
49. Abraham WT, Fisher WG, Smith AL, et al. Cardiac resynchronization in chronic heart failure. N Engl J Med. 2002;346:1845–53.
50. Bristow MR, Saxon LA, Boehmer J, et al. Cardiac-resynchronization therapy with or without an implantable defibrillator in advanced chronic heart failure. N Engl J Med. 2004;350:2140–50.
51. Cleland JG, Daubert JC, Erdmann E, et al. The effect of cardiac resynchronization on morbidity and mortality in heart failure. N Engl J Med. 2005;352:1539–49.
52. Moss AJ, Hall WJ, Cannom DS, et al. Cardiac-resynchronization therapy for the prevention of heart-failure events. N Engl J Med. 2009;361:1329–38.
53. Tang AS, Wells GA, Talajic M, et al. Cardiac-resynchronization therapy for mild-to-moderate heart failure. N Engl J Med. 2010;363:2385–95.
54. Zile MR, Baicu CF, Gaasch WH. Diastolic heart failure – abnormalities in active relaxation and passive stiffness of the left ventricle. N Engl J Med. 2004;350:1953–9.
55. Kasner M, Westermann D, Steendijk P, et al. Utility of Doppler echocardiography and tissue Doppler imaging in the estimation of diastolic function in heart failure with normal ejection fraction: a comparative Doppler-conductance catheterization study. Circulation. 2007;116: 637–47.
56. Yusuf S, Pfeffer MA, Swedberg K, et al. Effects of candesartan in patients with chronic heart failure and preserved left-ventricular ejection fraction: the CHARM-Preserved Trial. Lancet. 2003;362:777–81.
57. Massie BM, Carson PE, McMurray JJ, et al. Irbesartan in patients with heart failure and preserved ejection fraction. N Engl J Med. 2008;359:2456–67.
58. Andrew P. Diastolic heart failure demystified. Chest. 2003;124:744–53.

# Chapter 6
# Valvular Diseases

## Aortic Stenosis

### Etiology and Pathophysiology

Aortic stenosis (AS) occurs when there is obstruction of blood flow across the aortic valve. AS can result from a congenitally abnormal valve, rheumatic fever, or degenerative/calcific disease. The incidence of the various etiologies differs according to age at presentation. In children, AS generally results from a congenital abnormality. This is either a supravalvular or subvalvular obstruction, or occasionally valvular stenosis, usually in the form of a unicuspid valve in which two of the three commissures are fused, resulting in obstruction and symptoms in infancy.

Bicuspid aortic valve is the most common congenital heart defect, occurring in 2% of the population with a male predominance and familial clustering [1]. A bicuspid aortic valve tends to thicken and calcify, with symptoms of AS usually occurring in the third to fifth decade of life [2].

In aortic stenosis due to rheumatic heart disease there is also commissural fusion, but symptoms tend to develop later in life, usually in the fifth or sixth decade. Degenerative AS, on the other hand, is a senile calcific disease of the aortic valve leaflets and not the commissures, leading to progressive restriction of leaflet mobility. The histological features of calcific AS are similar to those seen in atherosclerosis [3]. The prevalence of AS increases with age, affecting 1.3% of people aged 65–74, and 4% of people above the age of 85.

Aortic sclerosis is the term used to describe thickening and calcification of the aortic valve without restriction of motion. The prevalence of aortic sclerosis also increases with age, affecting with 20% of people aged 65–74, and 48% above age 85 [4, 5]. Risk factors for developing aortic sclerosis include age, smoking, elevated LDL and lipoprotein A levels, diabetes mellitus, hypertension, and male sex [5]. An echocardiographic study showed that 16% of patients with aortic sclerosis progress

S. Hollenberg and S. Heitner, *Cardiology in Family Practice: A Practical Guide*, 113
Current Clinical Practice 1, DOI 10.1007/978-1-61779-385-1_6,
© Springer Science+Business Media, LLC 2012

to develop AS [6]. Aortic sclerosis by itself carries a slightly increased risk of cardiovascular morbidity and mortality [3].

As obstruction to left ventricular outflow increases, a greater left ventricular driving pressure is required to maintain stroke volume. This in turn results in an increase in wall stress (pressure×radius/wall thickness by the Laplace principle). Left ventricular hypertrophy ensues as a compensatory mechanism to reduce wall stress. This hypertrophy leads to a decrease in left ventricular compliance and diastolic dysfunction. Increased wall stress and LV mass also increase myocardial oxygen demand, and this, in combination with decreased aortic pressures as a result of the outflow obstruction can cause subendocardial ischemia and chest pain.

## Clinical Features

Patients with AS may remain relatively asymptomatic, even as obstruction progresses. The hypertrophied heart can often generate the very high intraventricular pressures necessary for the maintenance of a normal stroke volume. The first symptoms usually occur as a result of the diastolic dysfunction, but clinical manifestations of decreases in cardiac output and coronary blood flow eventually ensue. Patients may experience dyspnea, angina, and exertional syncope. Once symptomatic AS is present, the untreated mortality is quite high, with average survival less than 2–3 years.

The classical physical findings include a delayed and diminished carotid upstroke (*pulsus parvus et tardus*), a harsh systolic ejection murmur that increases with inspiration and radiates up the carotid arteries, and signs of left ventricular hypertrophy. The intensity of the murmur is not necessarily a reliable index of the severity of stenosis since the murmur may actually get softer as the left ventricle begins to fail and cardiac output diminishes. The murmur, however, does tend peak later in systole with increasing severity of the AS.

If the valve leaflets are still mobile, a systolic ejection click may be audible, and this implies less severe AS. The second heart sound may be soft as a result of decreased leaflet excursion, and there may be paradoxical splitting of $S_2$ due to prolongation of the LV ejection time. An $S_4$ may result from decreased LV compliance, and heart failure may produce an $S_3$ gallop.

The ECG most often shows left ventricular hypertrophy, often with a strain pattern. Extensive calcifications can result in intraventricular conduction delay. Chest radiography may show aortic calcifications and rounding of the left ventricular apex in addition to cardiomegaly.

Doppler echocardiography is generally the most accessible and useful diagnostic modality used in the workup of suspected AS. Echocardiography can reliably assess LV size and function, valvular morphology, transvalvular pressure gradients, and allow for calculation of valvular area, giving the clinician a good idea of the overall severity of the stenosis [7]. Importantly, one should always be aware that the transvalvular gradient may in fact be lower than expected in patients with depressed left ventricular function and decreased cardiac output; use of area to assess the severity of valvular stenosis is usually preferable. Careful dobutamine infusion with measurement of cardiac output and valvular gradient can help differentiate between low-output severe AS and non-significant stenosis.

The normal aortic valve area is 3–4 cm². Severity is graded by valve area and transvalvular gradient into mild, moderate, and severe (Table 6.1). Patients with mild AS should get an echocardiogram every 3–5 years, moderate AS every 1–2 years, and severe AS annually [8, 9]. Echocardiography should also be performed whenever there is a clinical change in patient status. Cardiac catheterization is needed to only confirm the severity of the AS only in the setting of a non-diagnostic echocardiogram. Coronary angiography, however, is frequently done prior to valve surgery as an accurate means of assessing the need for synchronous coronary artery bypass grafting. Exercise testing should not be done in patients with symptomatic AS. Substantial data support the use of exercise testing in asymptomatic severe aortic stenosis, when supervised by an experienced physician. This has been shown to be useful as a predictor for future events, as well as a useful tool for unmasking symptomatic aortic stenosis in patients who have gradually adjusted their lives to accommodate decreasing stroke volumes [10].

**Table 6.1** Classification of aortic stenosis

|          | Aortic valve area (cm³) | Transvalvular gradient (mmHg) |
|----------|-------------------------|-------------------------------|
| Mild     | >1.5                    | 25                            |
| Moderate | 1.0–1.5                 | 25–40                         |
| Severe   | <1.0                    | >40                           |

## *Treatment*

There is no effective medical therapy to relieve obstruction in patients with AS. Initial suggestions that intensive lipid-lowering therapy with statins may reduce progression [11, 12], have not been validated in larger clinical trials [13]. Vasodilators and diuretics should be used with extreme caution in these patients, since hypotension can lead to myocardial ischemia, decreasing systolic function and cardiac output with worsening hypotension – setting up a downward spiral that is very difficult to break. Asymptomatic patients should be counseled regarding physical activity. The ACC/AHA guidelines recommend that asymptomatic patients with mild AS can participate in some competitive sports, but patients with moderate or severe AS should avoid competitive sports [8]. Antimicrobial prophylaxis is no longer routinely advised for patients with valvular heart disease, including AS, undergoing dental, gastrointestinal, or genitourinary procedures [14].

Aortic valve replacement surgery is the current gold standard for treatment in symptomatic AS [8]. Patients with severe AS who are asymptomatic should also be considered for aortic valve replacement if they have LV systolic dysfunction (ejection fraction <50%), hypotension or symptoms during exercise, or a valve area <0.6 cm² with perioperative mortality is expected to be less than 1% [8]. Patients with moderate AS who are undergoing cardiac surgery for other reasons, should be considered for concomitant aortic valve replacement even in the absence of symptoms.

A more contemporary non-surgical technology is currently being evaluated and shows tremendous promise. Transcatheter aortic valve implantation (TAVI) was recently shown to be very effective in reducing symptoms and mortality in patients deemed to be unsuitable for surgical valve replacement [15]. Randomized studies comparing this technology to the standard surgical approach are ongoing.

Patient age, comorbidities, and preference need to be taken in to account when selecting between a mechanical prosthesis (longer durability but requires long-term anticoagulation) and a bioprosthetic valve (shorter durability but no need for long-term anticoagulation).

## Aortic Regurgitation

### Etiology and Pathophysiology

Aortic regurgitation (AR) is caused either by malcoaptation of the aortic valve leaflets or perforation of the individual leaflets. Malcoaptation occurs as a result of primary abnormalities of the aortic leaflets themselves, or the aortic root.

Acute AR may result from endocarditis, trauma, dissection of the aortic root, rupture of a sinus of Valsalva or of a myxomatous valve cusp, and acute dysfunction of a prosthetic valve.

In acute AR, the incompetent aortic valve causes acute volume overload and consequent diastolic pressure overload of the left ventricle (LV). The LV is unable to compensate for the increase in volume by increasing the end-diastolic volume, and subsequent rapid elevations are seen in the left ventricular end-diastolic and left atrial pressures. Furthermore, the effective stroke volume is decreased as a result of the backward displacement of blood volume during ventricular diastole (regurgitant fraction). In an effort to maintain an adequate forward cardiac output, a compensatory tachycardia ensues, although in acute and severe AR, this may not be sufficient and pulmonary edema with cardiogenic shock results.

Chronic AR is usually due to a progressive deterioration of the aortic leaflets or root. Causes range from a bicuspid valve, rheumatic heart disease, endocarditis, Marfan's syndrome, connective tissue diseases, syphilis, and hypertension.

Chronic AR is generally well tolerated because the left ventricle has time to dilate in response to the chronic volume overload produced by the regurgitant volume. This compensatory response increases forward stroke volume and maintains effective cardiac output. Over time the left ventricle dilates and hypertrophies, but at the terminal capabilities of this compensatory mechanism, LV end-diastolic and left atrial pressure increase, and symptoms may ensue.

## Clinical Features

Early in chronic AR, patients are usually relatively asymptomatic with occasional vague complaints of fatigue and palpitations. The usual presenting symptom is dyspnea.

Classic auscultatory signs of chronic AR include a soft $S_2$ in addition to the blowing decrescendo diastolic murmur, which is best heard with the patient leaning forward during end expiration. A systolic flow murmur is frequently audible as well. $P_2$ may be loud if the patient has developed pulmonary hypertension. Rapid left ventricular filling may produce a third heart sound. Severe AR may cause mitral valve preclosure and an apical diastolic murmur of relative MS across a structurally normal valve (Austin Flint murmur).

The peripheral signs of severe chronic AR include a wide pulse pressure (Corrigan's pulse), systolic head bobbing (Demusset sign), systolic pulsations of the uvula (Mueller's sign), pistol shot pulses (Traube sign), capillary pulsations (Quicke's pulses), to-and-fro femoral bruits (Duroziez's sign), and Hills sign (lower extremity blood pressure greater than upper extremity BP).

In acute AR, many of the characteristic physical findings of chronic AR are often less impressive or absent. Pulse pressure may not be increased because systolic pressure is reduced and the aortic diastolic pressure equilibrates with the elevated LV diastolic pressure, but tachycardia is invariably present. Due to equilibration between the aortic and ventricular diastolic pressure, the diastolic murmur may be short and soft or even inaudible. Mitral valve preclosure may produce a soft $S_1$.

In chronic AR, chest radiography shows cardiomegaly, with or without signs of pulmonary vascular congestion. The aortic root may be dilated. In acute AR, cardiomegaly may be absent on chest X-ray, but pulmonary edema is usual. Similarly, the EKG in chronic AR will show left ventricular hypertrophy, often with nonspecific ST-T changes of LV strain, and left atrial enlargement. In acute AR only sinus tachycardia and nonspecific ST changes may be present.

Echocardiography is the most useful technique for the diagnosis and assessment of severity in both acute and chronic AR. Two-dimensional echocardiography can be used to assess chamber and aortic root size, left ventricular function, as well as delineate the etiology. If aortic dissection or endocarditis with aortic ring abscess is suspected, transesophageal echocardiography is recommended. Doppler echocardiography can reliably define the severity of the AR. Left ventricular dimensions and systolic performance are important criteria used in the decision about timing of surgical intervention [8]. Cardiac catheterization is rarely needed for the confirmation of the severity of the regurgitation, but is generally indicated in patients at risk of coronary atherosclerosis for preoperative assessment of coronary artery disease.

## Treatment

Acute severe AR is a surgical emergency that often presents with cardiogenic shock. An attempt should be made to stabilize patients medically prior to surgery. Diuretics and intravenous nitrates are useful at reducing preload, and sodium nitroprusside or ACE inhibitors are good choices for afterload reduction, if the blood pressure permits [16]. Inotropic agents such a dopamine or dobutamine may be necessary to support cardiac output and temporarily lower left ventricular end-diastolic pressure until surgical intervention can be performed. Intra-aortic balloon counterpulsation is contraindicated in patients with AR. It should be remembered that tachycardia is compensatory and the use of beta blocker is relatively contraindicated given that any decrease in heart rate results in an increase in diastolic filling time and subsequently increases the regurgitant volume. With that said, cautious use of beta blockers may be indicated in acute severe AR associated with type A aortic dissection

In chronic severe AR, chronic therapy with vasodilators, such as ACE inhibitors, nifedipine, or hydralazine can reduce left ventricular end-diastolic volume and mass, and maintain ejection fraction [8, 17, 18]. Vasodilator use should be limited to symptomatic patients, patients with increased left ventricular volume but normal systolic function, and in patients with decompensated heart failure as a means to hemodynamic stabilization prior to surgical intervention. No benefit has been shown for vasodilator use as means to delay progression of mild or moderate AR, ventricular dysfunction or the development of symptoms in asymptomatic patients with normal ventricular volumes [8]. Nifedipine has however been documented to delay the need for aortic valve replacement in asymptomatic patients with severe AR [18].

Vigilant clinical assessment of asymptomatic patients with AR is recommended with serial clinical assessments and echocardiography every 6–12 months. Patients with severe AR should be advised to avoid isometric exercises. Asymptomatic patients can participate in most forms of physical activity, including competitive sports, but all patients with AR are advised to avoid isometric exercise. Prophylaxis against bacterial endocarditis is no longer routinely recommended [14].

Aortic valve replacement is recommended in all patients with symptomatic AR, irrespective of left ventricular performance. Asymptomatic patients with left ventricular dysfunction or significant dilatation should also undergo valve replacement. Asymptomatic patients with moderate or severe AR who are undergoing cardiac surgery for other reasons should also be considered candidates for valve replacement. Patient age, comorbidities, and preference need to be taken in to account in the decision about a mechanical prosthesis (longer durability but requires long-term anticoagulation) vs. a bioprosthetic valve (shorter durability but no need for long-term anticoagulation).

## Mitral Stenosis

### Etiology and Pathophysiology

Mitral stenosis (MS) is a narrowing of the mitral valve that impedes blood flow from the left atrium to the left ventricle during diastole. The most common cause of MS is rheumatic fever, although a history of rheumatic fever is frequently not obtained.

There is a latency period of about 10–20 years before the patient develops symptoms of mitral stenosis. Less common etiologies of left ventricular inflow obstruction include atrial myxoma, carcinoid, congenital MS, systemic lupuserythematosis, rheumatoid arthritis, and the mucopolysacharroidoses.

The normal mitral valve orifice area is 4–6 cm², with symptoms rarely developing before the valve area decreases below 2.5 cm² [19]. A valve area >2 cm² is considered mildly stenotic, between 1 and 2 cm² is moderate, and <1 cm² is severe MS (see Table 6.2). As the valve area decreases, the LA pressure rises in an effort to maintain left ventricular filling and cardiac output. The increase in LA pressure subsequently results in increased pressure in the pulmonary vasculature. Acute elevations in left atrial pressure tend to cause pulmonary edema. In rheumatic MS, the slowly progressive decrease in mitral valve orifice area results in a gradual increase in the necessary filling pressures. The pulmonary vasculature protects against the development of pulmonary edema by decreasing capillary permeability and this in turn, results in pulmonary hypertension. The end result is that patients may have impressively elevated left atrial and pulmonary arterial pressures at the time of diagnosis, without ever having developed pulmonary edema.

**Table 6.2** Classification of mitral stenosis (Adapted from: Bonow et al. [8])

|  | Mitral valve area (cm³) |
|---|---|
| Mild | >2.0 |
| Moderate | 1.0–2.0 |
| Severe | <1.0 |

It is important to appreciate that in order to allow the passage of blood across the stenotic valve, the diastolic filling period needs to be kept as long as possible. Any condition that results in tachycardia will shorten the diastolic filling time and cause acute elevation in left atrial pressure. This explains why many patients with mitral stenosis tend to present with dyspnea and pulmonary edema after exercise, emotional stress, infection, pregnancy, or atrial fibrillation with a rapid ventricular response [20].

The left ventricle is generally protected in isolated MS. If the valve becomes sufficiently stenotic, LV filling and end-diastolic volume can diminish, leading to a decrease in stroke volume and cardiac output.

## Clinical Features

The initial symptom in MS is usually exertional dyspnea. Other symptoms include hemoptysis, orthopnea, paroxysmal nocturnal dyspnea, fatigue, palpitations, and thromboembolic events. In fact, thromboembolism due to atrial fibrillation may be the first manifestation of MS.

On physical examination, the first heart sound is loud because of increased left atrial pressure prior to mitral valve closure. A mid-diastolic opening snap may be heard as the LV pressure falls below the LA pressure and the mitral valve opens vigorously under the high filling pressure. As the severity of the MS increases and the left atrial pressure rises, the opening snap tends to move closer to $S_2$. The classic murmur of MS is a low-pitched mid-diastolic rumble, best appreciated at the apex of the heart with the patient lying in the left lateral position. Other signs of severe MS are referable to pulmonary hypertension, and include a loud $P_2$, jugular venous distension with a prominent a wave, and a right ventricular heave.

The classic ECG findings of MS are a broad notched P-wave (P mitrale) indicative of left atrial enlargement. Atrial fibrillation is also frequently present. As the patient develops pulmonary hypertension and right ventricular hypertrophy, the QRS axis shifts to the right with tall R waves in leads $V_1$ and $V_2$. Chest radiography in MS shows straightening of the left heart border, pulmonary venous congestion and dilated pulmonary arteries. As the left atrium enlarges posteriorly, it may compress the esophagus causing dysphagia, or stretch the recurrent laryngeal nerve and cause hoarseness (Ortner's syndrome).

Echocardiography is the definitive and essential diagnostic test and defines the valve anatomy, classifies the severity of the MS, and helps with the choice of treatment modalities. Doppler echocardiography can measure the transmitral gradient, mitral valve area, and the pulmonary artery pressure, which provide important information for evaluation of an asymptomatic patient. Morphologic evaluation of the mitral valve and subvalvular apparatus allow appropriate selection of patients for percutaneous mitral balloon valvuloplasty vs. mitral valve replacement [21].

## Therapy

MS is an obstructive condition, and as such medical therapies will palliate symptoms, but do nothing for the disease progression itself. When symptoms do occur, medical therapy can be very effective for symptom relief, but one should always consider relieving the obstruction via either interventional or surgical techniques. Diuretics are beneficial for symptoms associated with pulmonary vascular congestion and can be prescribed on an as-needed basis. Since exertional dyspnea usually results from increased heart rate, beta blockers or non-dihydropyridine calcium channel blockers can help prevent tachycardia and provide symptomatic relief by increasing diastolic filling time. Atrial fibrillation is poorly tolerated in MS as a result of both the rapid ventricular response rate as well as the loss of the atrial contraction necessary for left ventricular filling. Cardioversion should be considered, but if unsuccessful, digoxin, beta blockers, or calcium channel blockers, are useful in controlling the ventricular response rate.

Anticoagulation, unless contraindicated, should be given to all patients with MS and atrial fibrillation (paroxysmal and permanent) or to patients with a prior embolic event even if there is no direct evidence of an atrial arrhythmia [8]. There is also evidence to support the use of long-term anticoagulants in patients thought to be at risk of atrial fibrillation (left atrial size >5.5 cm on echocardiography) [22]. The target INR should be 2.5, with a range from 2 to 3. If a patient has an embolic event while on anticoagulation, aspirin (75–100 mg/day) is usually added, and the target INR is increased to 3.0 (range 2.5–3.5). If the patient can not tolerate aspirin, clopidogrel 75 mg/day can be substituted [22].

Asymptomatic patients with mild MS need to be followed annually with a history, physical exam, ECG, and chest X-ray. Echocardiography is recommended at the initial presentation and thereafter, if there is a change in clinical status. If patients have palpitations, then ambulatory ECG monitoring is recommended to rule out paroxysmal atrial fibrillation. Patients with severe MS should be followed with a clinical exam every 6 months and echocardiography every 12 months. Patients with severe MS can be asymptomatic due to adjustments in lifestyle and therefore these patients should be evaluated by echocardiography to measure pulmonary arterial pressures. Bacterial endocarditis prophylaxis is no longer recommended routinely for patients with MS [14]. Physical exercise should be limited in patients with moderate to severe MS.

Guidelines for interventional therapy, surgical repair, or valve replacement have been promulgated by the ACC/AHA. Valvotomy is recommended for asymptomatic patients with moderate or severe MS with pulmonary artery pressure >50 mmHg or poor exercise tolerance, symptomatic patients with moderate to severe MS, or symptomatic patients with mild MS and increased pulmonary artery pressure. Contraindications to valvotomy are unsuitable anatomy, left atrial thrombus, and moderate to severe MR. Surgical repair is recommended for symptomatic patients with moderate to severe MS, if balloon valvotomy is not available or anatomically possible, and in the presence left atrial thrombus. Selection of a bioprosthetic or mechanical valve takes into consideration patient age, comorbidities, and preference.

# Mitral Regurgitation

## Etiology and Pathophysiology

Mitral regurgitation (MR) can be acute or chronic; both the presentations and etiologies differ. Acute MR may result from chordal rupture in patients with myxomatous valves, acute infective endocarditis, blunt or penetrating chest trauma, and papillary muscle rupture or dysfunction in the setting of inferior infarction. Chronic MR occurs in the setting of mitral valve prolapse, rheumatic heart disease, infectious endocarditis, collagen vascular disease, dilated cardiomyopathy, and mitral annular calcification.

In acute MR, the sudden increase in left atrial volume as a result of the regurgitant blood from the left ventricle results in an increase in left atrial pressure and subsequently acute pulmonary edema. Left ventricular ejection into the lower-pressure left atrium impairs forward flow through the aortic valve, which leads to a lower cardiac output and potentially cardiogenic shock.

In chronic MR, compensatory dilation of the left atrium increases its capacity and decreases LA pressure. The left ventricle compensates for its volume overload by eccentric hypertrophy and dilation, helping to maintain cardiac output. Eventually the increased volume can increase LV wall stress and impair ventricular performance. It is important to recognize that ejection fraction is not a reliable measure of ventricular performance in MR, because left ventricular ejection occurs through both the aortic valve and the low-pressure mitral valve. As such, the parameters used to time Intervention may sometimes be appropriate even with a seemingly normal left ventricular ejection fraction.

## Clinical Features

Patients with acute severe MR usually presents dramatically with flash pulmonary edema, hypotension, and cardiogenic shock. The murmur of acute MR may be limited to early systole because of rapid equalization of pressures in the left atrium and left ventricle. Importantly, the murmur may be soft or inaudible, especially when cardiac output is low.

Chronic MR, on the other hand, is generally well tolerated, and patients may remain asymptomatic for years. Over time, as the left ventricle enlarges, patients may present with heart failure symptoms, such as fatigue, dyspnea, orthopnea, and edema.

On physical examination the apical impulse is hyperkinetic and displaced laterally in chronic MR. A holosystolic apical murmur that usually radiates to the axilla can be auscultated, sometimes with a palpable systolic thrill; an $S_3$ is frequently present. In patients with mitral valve prolapse, a mid-systolic click may be heard. With the development of pulmonary hypertension, jugular venous pressure is elevated and the pulmonary component of the second heart sound is loud. A right ventricle heave may be present as well.

The electrocardiogram usually reflects the anatomical changes in the heart with evidence of left ventricular hypertrophy, left atrial enlargement, and possibly atrial fibrillation. The chest radiograph will show cardiomegaly, with or without pulmonary congestion. The pulmonary arteries may be dilated. In acute MR, pulmonary edema is evident.

Echocardiography is very useful in delineating the severity and often the etiology of the MR (structural vs. functional MR). Echocardiography is used to define the mitral valve morphology, identify chordal and papillary muscle pathology, and measure the degree of annular dilatation and left atrial size. Doppler echocardiography is a reliable means of classifying the severity of the MR and is also useful in the estimation of pulmonary artery pressures. Overall left ventricular function and end-systolic dimensions are critical in the timing of potential operative repair or replacement. Transesophageal echocardiography is very useful prior to surgery to assist the surgeon in the decision of whether to attempt mitral valve repair versus replacement.

Cardiac catheterization with ventriculography can help confirm the severity of MR, but is generally used to assess the degree of coronary artery disease prior to surgery or in suspected ischemic MR.

## Therapy

Management of acute severe mitral regurgitation entails stabilization of the patient with intravenous afterload reduction (nitroprusside or enalaprilat) and intra-aortic balloon counterpulsation, but these are only temporizing measures. Inotropic or vasopressor support may also be necessary to assist with hemodynamic stabilization. Nitrates may be incorporated if ischemia is causing or contributing to acute MR. Definitive therapy remains surgical valve repair or replacement, which should be undertaken urgently since clinical deterioration can be sudden.

Asymptomatic patients with mild MR without pulmonary hypertension, left ventricular dysfunction or dilatation should be followed annually. Echocardiography should be done initially and repeated if there is a change in clinical status. Patients with moderate MR should have an annual exam and echocardiography. Asymptomatic patients with severe MR should be followed every 6–12 months with a clinical exam and echocardiography [8].

Chronic vasodilatory therapy is indicated for asymptomatic patients with MR, only if there is comorbidity such as hypertension, left ventricular dysfunction, or myocardial ischemia. Patients with symptomatic mitral regurgitation, or those with left ventricular dysfunction, however, do benefit from vasodilators [23]. In these patients, therapy with ACE inhibitors and beta blockers, along with biventricular pacing when indicated, has been shown to decrease the severity of functional MR [24, 25]. Diuretics and digoxin are used as needed for the symptoms of heart failure. Bacterial endocarditis prophylaxis is no longer recommended routinely for all patients with MR [14].

Surgery is recommended for all symptomatic patients with acute severe MR. As a general rule, one should expect some degree of a decrease in left ventricular systolic function after surgical therapy for MR. With this in mind, surgery is most suitable in patients with chronic severe MR in the absence of severe LV systolic dysfunction (EF >30%) or significant LV dilatation (LV end-systolic dimension of greater than 5.5 cm). It is currently recommended that surgery be considered in both symptomatic and asymptomatic patients with severe MR and left ventricular end-systolic dimension >45 mm or ejection fraction less than 55–60% (but greater than 30%) [26]. Mitral valve repair is the procedure of choice when the valve morphology is amenable to repair. Most clinicians lower their threshold for operative intervention when valve repair is felt to be feasible. Mitral valve repair tends to be associated with a lesser decrement in post-operative LV systolic function.

Asymptomatic patients with ejection fractions >60% and normal left ventricular dimensions should be followed clinically and with serial echocardiography annually (Fig. 6.1) [9].

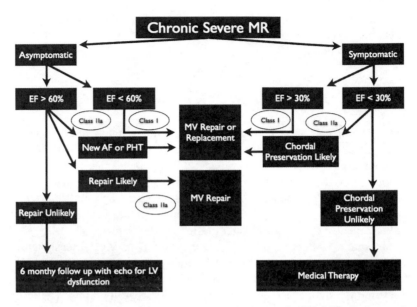

**Fig. 6.1** Algorithm for treatment of chronic severe mitral regurgitation. *MR* mitral regurgitation; *AF* atrial fibrillation; *PHT* pulmonary hypertension. *LV* left ventricle; *EF* ejection fraction

Should mitral valve sparing surgery not be feasible, mitral valve replacement is a second option, with either chordal sparing or chordal reconstruction, both of which help to preserve left ventricular geometry. A variety of factors need to be considered when selecting the type of valve prosthesis (age, comorbidities, patient preference, and ability to remain of long-term anticoagulation).

## Tricuspid Valve Disease

### *Etiology and Pathophysiology*

Tricuspid Regurgitation (TR) and tricuspid stenosis (TS) occur very rarely in isolation. Over and above that, the morbidity and mortality linked with diseases of the tricuspid valve in isolation rarely justify the surgical risk associated with open-heart surgery.

On the whole, the majority of TR is functional in origin, most commonly related to elevations in right heart pressures. This in turn results in right ventricular (RV) enlargement, tricuspid annular dilatation, and consequent leaflet malcoaptation with regurgitation. RV hypertension occurs in MS, pulmonic valve stenosis, right ventricular infarction, dilated cardiomyopathy, and the various causes of pulmonary hypertension [27]. Pacemaker lead-induced functional TR to varying degrees is fairly common but treatment is rarely indicated. Structural abnormalities of the tricuspid valve occur with infective endocarditis, rheumatic valvulitis, carcinoid syndrome, rheumatoid arthritis, radiation therapy, trauma, Marfan syndrome with tricuspid valve prolapse, or congenital disorders such as Ebstein's anomaly.

TS is exceedingly rare, and when present is most likely rheumatic in origin. Other causes of TS include congenital abnormalities, carcinoid syndrome, Fabry's disease, Whipple's disease, and obstructive mass lesions (e.g., right atrial myxoma) [28].


## Diagnosis and Treatment

The clinical features of TS include signs of the associated valvulopathies seen in chronic rheumatic heart disease (MR, MS, TR, AS, and AR), a giant *a* wave on jugular vein examination, and a diastolic murmur that increases in intensity with inspiration, a finding that can be difficult to auscultate. The clinical features of TR include abnormal systolic *c* and *v* waves on jugular vein examination and a holosystolic murmur that increases with inspiration and is best heard over the lower left parasternal area. In severe TR there may be systolic hepatic pulsation [29]. Echocardiography is key to the diagnosis and grading of TR and TS [30].

Therapy for the tricuspid pathology is usually dictated by the comorbid valvulopathy (e.g., MS or MR). When indicated, surgery for TR should be valve-sparing (usually annuloplasty) if anatomically and technically feasible. If annuloplasty is not a possibility, then a bioprosthetic valve is most appropriate given the higher rate of valve thrombosis if a mechanical valve is used in the tricuspid position [31].

It is important to realize that although primary tricuspid valvulopathies are uncommon and are often less serious than the mitral or aortic counterparts, patients with severe TR of any cause tend to have a poor long-term outcome because of RV dysfunction and systemic venous congestion [32].


# References

1. Otto CM, Kuusisto J, Reichenbach DD, Gown AM, O'Brien KD. Characterization of the early lesion of 'degenerative' valvular aortic stenosis. Histological and immunohistochemical studies. Circulation. 1994;90:844–53.
2. Fenoglio Jr JJ, McAllister Jr HA, DeCastro CM, Davia JE, Cheitlin MD. Congenital bicuspid aortic valve after age 20. Am J Cardiol. 1977;39:164–9.
3. Otto CM, Lind BK, Kitzman DW, Gersh BJ, Siscovick DS. Association of aortic-valve sclerosis with cardiovascular mortality and morbidity in the elderly. N Engl J Med. 1999;341:142–7.
4. Lindroos M, Kupari M, Heikkila J, Tilvis R. Prevalence of aortic valve abnormalities in the elderly: an echocardiographic study of a random population sample. J Am Coll Cardiol. 1993;21:1220–5.
5. Stewart BF, Siscovick D, Lind BK, et al. Clinical factors associated with calcific aortic valve disease. Cardiovascular Health Study. J Am Coll Cardiol. 1997;29:630–4.

6. Cosmi JE, Kort S, Tunick PA, et al. The risk of the development of aortic stenosis in patients with "benign" aortic valve thickening. Arch Intern Med. 2002;162:2345–7.

7. Cheitlin MD, Armstrong WF, Aurigemma GP, et al. ACC/AHA/ASE 2003 guideline update for the clinical application of echocardiography: summary article: a report of the American College of Cardiology/American Heart Association Task Force on Practice Guidelines (ACC/AHA/ASE Committee to Update the 1997 Guidelines for the Clinical Application of Echocardiography). Circulation. 2003;108:1146–62.

8. Bonow RO, Carabello BA, Chatterjee K, et al. ACC/AHA 2006 guidelines for the management of patients with valvular heart disease: a report of the American College of Cardiology/American Heart Association Task Force on Practice Guidelines (writing Committee to Revise the 1998 guidelines for the management of patients with valvular heart disease) developed in collaboration with the Society of Cardiovascular Anesthesiologists endorsed by the Society for Cardiovascular Angiography and Interventions and the Society of Thoracic Surgeons. J Am Coll Cardiol. 2006;48:e1–148.

9. Bonow RO, Carabello B, De Leon Jr AC. et al. Guidelines for the management of patients with valvular heart disease: executive summary. A report of the American College of Cardiology/American Heart Association Task Force on Practice Guidelines (Committee on Management of Patients with Valvular Heart Disease). Circulation. 1998;98:1949–84.

10. Das P, Rimington H, Chambers J. Exercise testing to stratify risk in aortic stenosis. Eur Heart J. 2005;26:1309–13.

11. Rosenhek R, Rader F, Loho N, et al. Statins but not angiotensin-converting enzyme inhibitors delay progression of aortic stenosis. Circulation. 2004;110:1291–5.

12. Bellamy MF, Pellikka PA, Klarich KW, Tajik AJ, Enriquez-Sarano M. Association of cholesterol levels, hydroxymethylglutaryl coenzyme-A reductase inhibitor treatment, and progression of aortic stenosis in the community. J Am Coll Cardiol. 2002;40:1723–30.

13. Cowell SJ, Newby DE, Prescott RJ, et al. A randomized trial of intensive lipid-lowering therapy in calcific aortic stenosis. N Engl J Med. 2005;352:2389–97.

14. Wilson W, Taubert KA, Gewitz M, et al. Prevention of infective endocarditis: guidelines from the American Heart Association: a guideline from the American Heart Association Rheumatic Fever, Endocarditis, and Kawasaki Disease Committee, Council on Cardiovascular Disease in the Young, and the Council on Clinical Cardiology, Council on Cardiovascular Surgery and Anesthesia, and the Quality of Care and Outcomes Research Interdisciplinary Working Group. Circulation. 2007;116:1736–54.

15. Leon MB, Smith CR, Mack M, et al. Transcatheter aortic-valve implantation for aortic stenosis in patients who cannot undergo surgery. N Engl J Med. 2010;363:1597–607.

16. Khan SS, Gray RJ. Valvular emergencies. Cardiol Clin. 1991;9:689–709.

17. Lin M, Chiang HT, Lin SL, et al. Vasodilator therapy in chronic asymptomatic aortic regurgitation: enalapril versus hydralazine therapy. J Am Coll Cardiol. 1994;24:1046–53.

18. Scognamiglio R, Rahimtoola SH, Fasoli G, Nistri S, Dalla Volta S. Nifedipine in asymptomatic patients with severe aortic regurgitation and normal left ventricular function. N Engl J Med. 1994;331:689–94.

19. Gorlin R, Gorlin SG. Hydraulic formula for calculation of the area of stenotic mitral valve, other cardiac values and central circulatory shunts. Am Heart J. 1951;41:1–29.

20. Hugenholtz PG, Ryan TJ, Stein SW, Abelmann WH. The spectrum of pure mitral stenosis. Hemodynamic studies in relation to clinical disability. Am J Cardiol. 1962;10:773–84.

21. Wilkins GT, Weyman AE, Abascal VM, Block PC, Palacios IF. Percutaneous balloon dilatation of the mitral valve: an analysis of echocardiographic variables related to outcome and the mechanism of dilatation. Br Heart J. 1988;60:299–308.

22. Salem DN, Stein PD, Al-Ahmad A, et al. Antithrombotic therapy in valvular heart disease – native and prosthetic: the Seventh ACCP Conference on Antithrombotic and Thrombolytic Therapy. Chest. 2004;126:457S–82S.

23. Greenberg BH, DeMots H, Murphy E, Rahimtoola SH. Arterial dilators in mitral regurgitation: effects on rest and exercise hemodynamics and long-term clinical follow-up. Circulation. 1982;65:181–7.

24. Capomolla S, Febo O, Gnemmi M, et al. Beta-blockade therapy in chronic heart failure: diastolic function and mitral regurgitation improvement by carvedilol. Am Heart J. 2000;139:596–608.
25. Linde C, Leclercq C, Rex S, et al. Long-term benefits of biventricular pacing in congestive heart failure: results from the MUltisite STimulation in Cardiomyopathy (MUSTIC) study. J Am Coll Cardiol. 2002;40:111–8.
26. Enriquez-Sarano M, Schaff HV, Orszulak TA, Tajik AJ, Bailey KR, Frye RL. Valve repair improves the outcome of surgery for mitral regurgitation. A multivariate analysis. Circulation. 1995;91:1022–8.
27. Waller BF, Moriarty AT, Eble JN, Davey DM, Hawley DA, Pless JE. Etiology of pure tricuspid regurgitation based on anular circumference and leaflet area: analysis of 45 necropsy patients with clinical and morphologic evidence of pure tricuspid regurgitation. J Am Coll Cardiol. 1986;7:1063–74.
28. Waller BF, Howard J, Fess S. Pathology of tricuspid valve stenosis and pure tricuspid regurgitation – part I. Clin Cardiol. 1995;18:97–102.
29. Rivera JM, Vandervoort PM, Vazquez de Prada JA, et al. Vazquez de Prada JA, et al. Which physical factors determine tricuspid regurgitation jet area in the clinical setting? Am J Cardiol. 1993;72:1305–9.
30. Zoghbi WA, Enriquez-Sarano M, Foster E, et al. Recommendations for evaluation of the severity of native valvular regurgitation with two-dimensional and Doppler echocardiography. J Am Soc Echocardiogr. 2003;16:777–802.
31. Dreyfus GD, Corbi PJ, Chan KM, Bahrami T. Secondary tricuspid regurgitation or dilatation: which should be the criteria for surgical repair? Ann Thorac Surg. 2005;79:127–32.
32. Sagie A, Schwammenthal E, Newell JB, et al. Significant tricuspid regurgitation is a marker for adverse outcome in patients undergoing percutaneous balloon mitral valvuloplasty. J Am Coll Cardiol. 1994;24:696–702.

# Chapter 7
# Pericardial Diseases

## Acute Pericarditis

### Etiology and Pathophysiology

The pericardium is a fibroelastic sac that is made up of two layers (visceral and parietal), between which is contained 15–50°cc of fluid [1]. Acute pericarditis is the result of acute inflammation of the pericardium with or without associated pericardial effusion. About 90% of cases of acute pericarditis are idiopathic or viral; other causes include uremia, collagen vascular diseases, neoplasm, and inflammation after acute myocardial infarction or pericardial injury.

Acute pericarditis can also occur after a myocardial infarction or following cardiac surgery. Potential sequelae of acute pericarditis include cardiac tamponade and constrictive pericarditis.

### Clinical Features

Severe, retrosternal chest pain is the most common symptom of acute pericarditis. The pain is often sharp and pleuritic in nature, and may radiate to the shoulder, neck, and trapezius muscle ridges. The referred pain to the trapezius muscle ridges is due to irritation of the phrenic nerve as it transverses the pericardium [2]. The intensity of the pain can vary with position, often becoming worse when supine and improving when the patient leans forward. Pain is also commonly exacerbated by inspiration.

The classic physical sign is a pericardial friction rub. The rub is coarse in nature and usually best heard along the left sternal border and during breath holding. There

S. Hollenberg and S. Heitner, *Cardiology in Family Practice: A Practical Guide*, 129
Current Clinical Practice 1, DOI 10.1007/978-1-61779-385-1_7,
© Springer Science+Business Media, LLC 2012

are three components to this rub (triphasic), corresponding to the movement of the heart during atrial systole, ventricular systole and early ventricular diastole.

The diagnosis of pericarditis is usually made by electrocardiography, with diffuse ST elevation (usually not corresponding to an anatomic distribution, but this may not necessarily be the case in localized pericarditis) and PR segment depression. The electrocardiogram may show an evolution through four stages: Stage 1 – diffuse concave upsloping ST elevation and PR segment depression; Stage 2 – normalization of the ST and PR segments; Stage 3 – widespread T wave inversions; and Stage 4 – normalization of the T waves [3]. Stage 1 is observed in 80% of patients [4], but prompt initiation of therapy may prevent the appearance of all four stages [5]. On chest radiography, the cardiac silhouette may be entirely normal or may be enlarged if a pericardial effusion is present.

Mildly elevated plasma troponin levels can be observed in acute pericarditis. Troponin release is commonly associated with male gender, ST elevations, young age, and pericardial effusion, and generally resolves within 1 week after presentation [6]. The degree of troponin elevation is roughly related to the extent of myocardial inflammatory involvement and is not necessarily associated with a worse outcome [6].

Echocardiography can be used in patients with suspected pericarditis to evaluate for a pericardial effusion [7]. The absence of a pericardial effusion, however, does not exclude the diagnosis of acute pericarditis.

## *Therapy*

Treatment for acute pericarditis should be directed at the underlying cause. For patients with idiopathic pericarditis, the treatment should be directed at relieving the symptoms and decreasing the inflammation. Non-steroidal anti-inflammatory drugs, specifically ibuprofen, are recommended as the treatment of choice for acute pericarditis [8]. The dose of ibuprofen ranges from 300 to 800 mg every 6–8 h, depending on symptom severity and response to therapy. Indomethacin (50 mg TID) is also commonly employed. In postinfarction pericarditis, aspirin should be given at a dose of 650 mg every 4 h for 2–5 days [8]. Colchicine can also be used for symptomatic relief, either as monotherapy or in combination with non-steroidal agents [8]. Colchicine has also been shown in a randomized trial to reduce recurrence after an initial episode of acute pericarditis [9]. Steroids are recommended only for connective tissue disease, uremic pericarditis, and in selected cases of refractory pericarditis [8]. Importantly, there is developing evidence that although systemic corticosteroids effectively treat acute pericarditis, their use early in the disease may be associated with relapse after their taper [10]. To ensure resolution, patients should be followed up in the office setting. An echocardiogram is recommended if there is clinical suspicion of an effusion or if pericardial constriction is suspected [8].

Pericardiocentesis is indicated for tamponade, a high suspicion of purulent or neoplastic pericarditis, or for large or symptomatic effusions that persist despite medical therapy for more than 1 week [8].

# Cardiac Tamponade

## *Etiology and Pathophysiology*

Cardiac tamponade is a life-threatening condition that results from fluid accumulation in the pericardial space with an increase in intrapericardial pressure sufficient to alter cardiac filling. The right heart is usually most vulnerable to compression, owing to lower normal intracavitary pressures. The causes of tamponade are the same as the causes of pericardial effusions, and include pericarditis, malignancy, trauma, dissecting aortic aneurysm, tuberculosis, SLE, uremia and following surgical or invasive diagnostic procedures.

The pericardium normally has limited elasticity, and once the accumulation of fluid reaches the elastic capacity, pericardial pressure rises quickly. The consequences of pericardial fluid depend on the rate of accumulation, pericardial compliance, and patient blood volume. As little as 200 mL to as much as 2 L can cause tamponade [11]. Once the pericardium becomes inelastic, the heart and pericardial contents must compete for a fixed intrapericardial volume [12, 13].

Compensatory mechanisms that help maintain cardiac output ensue. These include increased right-sided filling pressures, tachycardia, increased ejection fraction, and increased peripheral vascular tone, all of which are mediated by increased sympathetic tone. With increasing intrapericardial pressure, there is less of a gradient between the atria and ventricles, resulting in slower intracardiac flow, lower volumes and cardiac output. The earliest echocardiographic evidence of tamponade physiology is seen during diastole, with compression of the right atrium and right ventricle. As the intrapericardial pressure increases further, the heart is compressed throughout the cardiac cycle. With inspiration, there is an increase in venous return and volume in the right ventricle, which causes the interventricular septum to bulge into the left ventricle, thus decreasing stroke volume, cardiac output, and blood pressure (pulsus paradoxus) [14]. With progression, blood pressure is decreased and cardiogenic shock ensues.

## *Clinical Features*

The symptoms of cardiac tamponade result from decreased cardiac output and pulmonary congestion. Symptoms can be dramatic, but are often non-specific, and include dyspnea, chest pain, weakness, orthopnea, cough, and dysphagia.

The classic physical examination findings are jugular venous distension, hypotension, and muffled heart sounds, known as Beck's triad. The jugular venous pulsations show a prominent $x$ (systolic) descent, and a markedly decreased or absent $y$ (diastolic) descent, reflecting impaired diastolic filling. Other findings include tachycardia, tachypnea, and pulsus paradoxus. Pulsus paradoxus is defined as a decrease in systolic blood greater than 10 mmHg pressure with inspiration, and results from increased right-sided filling with inspiration at the expense of left-sided filling, decreasing stroke volume. Pulsus paradoxus can also be seen in other conditions such as chronic obstructive pulmonary diseases, pulmonary embolism and hypovolemia. Hypotension is a late sign.

Findings on ECG associated with cardiac tamponade include low voltage and electrical alternans (changing electrical axis that results from swinging of the heart within the pericardial fluid). The ECG may show sinus tachycardia in the absence of any significant changes. The chest X-ray may show an enlarged cardiac silhouette ("water bottle" heart).

Echocardiography is indicated in all patients with suspected tamponade, not only to document the presence of a pericardial effusion but also to define its hemodynamic significance. Significant changes in transvalvular flow velocities with respiration are the echocardiographic equivalent of a pulsus paradoxus, and indicate that the effusion has hemodynamic impact. Inferior vena cava plethora is indicative of high venous pressures, and is the most sensitive, but least specific finding on echocardiography [15]. With tamponade, loss of the transmural pressure gradient in the right atrium and right ventricle can lead to diastolic collapse. Right ventricular collapse is more specific for tamponade than right atrial collapse [16, 17].

Cardiac tamponade is in essence a hemodynamic diagnosis that is made definitively by demonstration of elevation and equalization (within 5 mm of one another) of diastolic pressures in the right atrium, right ventricle, pulmonary artery, and pulmonary artery wedge pressure tracing, which entails right heart catheterization. Although echocardiographic evidence in the right clinical setting is often sufficient, right heart catheterization to measure pressures may be useful should diagnostic uncertainty remain.

## Therapy

Fluid therapy and vasopressor support are temporizing measures in patients with cardiac tamponade. The heart is maximally stimulated by sympathetic drive, and exogenous inotropic agents add little [14]. Definitive therapy requires removal of pericardial fluid either via pericardiocentesis or surgically.

Patients with tamponade physiology should be considered for emergent pericardiocentesis. Because of the inelasticity of the pericardium, hemodynamic relief can be obtained with the removal of only a relatively small amount of fluid. A multihole pigtail drainage catheter is usually left in place for 24 h for more complete drainage of pericardial fluid [14].

Pericardiocentesis is usually not effective in patients who are actively accumulating intrapericardial fluid, such as those with penetrating cardiac wounds, ruptured ventricular aneurysms, or aortic dissection [7]. In these patients emergent surgical correction is obviously required. A surgical approach is also preferred when a pericardial biopsy is required, if there are complex loculations, or for recurrent effusions [14].

# Constrictive Pericarditis

## Etiology and Pathophysiology

Pericardial constriction is the result of a thickened, scarred, sometimes calcified pericardium limiting cardiac volume. The scarring and inelasticity interferes with diastolic filling and ultimately decreases cardiac output. Constrictive pericarditis can occur after any pericardial disease. Most cases are idiopathic, and are probably result from chronic pericarditis. Tuberculous pericarditis eventually resulting in constriction is very common throughout the developing world, but is a much less common cause in the United States. Other etiologies include radiation, post-pericardotomy, malignancy, uremia, post-traumatic and connective tissue disorders.

The rigid pericardium restricts ventricular filling during diastole. Initially there is early rapid unrestricted filling that abruptly ceases at the end of the first third of diastole, resulting in the characteristic pericardial knock heard on examination. The hemodynamic hallmark of pericardial constriction is equalization of end-diastolic pressures in the four cardiac chambers. Stroke volume and cardiac output subsequently decrease, resulting in both left and right heart failure.

Other characteristic hemodynamic findings include a dip and plateau "square root" sign on the right ventricular pressure (which reflects the early rapid diastolic filling with sudden cessation). On the venous pressure tracing, the $a$ and $v$ waves are prominent and the $x$ and $y$ descents are steep, producing an M or W configuration. With the total cardiac volume fixed, the normal intrathoracic pressure changes seen during respiration are shielded from the heart by the pericardium. On the other hand, pressures in the pulmonary and systemic venous systems are affected by respiration. This phenomenon results in a paradoxical rise in the jugular venous pressure with inspiration and is termed "Kussmaul's" sign.

Pericardial constriction presents insidiously. Dyspnea on exertion, decreased exercise tolerance, and fatigue are usually the first symptoms. Other symptoms may include nonspecific abdominal symptoms and weight loss. As the constriction progresses, dyspnea worsens.

Patients with constrictive pericarditis present with manifestations of elevated systemic venous pressures and low cardiac output. There is marked jugular venous distension, hepatic congestion, ascites, and peripheral edema despite clear lungs. Other physical findings include Kussmaul's sign, and mid-diastolic pericardial knock, prominent $x$ and $y$ descents on examination of the jugular venous waveform. The characteristic auscultatory finding is a mid-diastolic pericardial knock, which represents a sudden cessation in ventricular inflow.

There are no specific findings on ECG for constrictive pericarditis, but low voltage, and T wave inversion or flattening may be seen. Chest radiograph may show pericardial calcifications, biatrial enlargement and pleural effusions.

Echocardiography with Doppler should be performed on all patients suspected of having constrictive pericarditis [7]. Echocardiographic features of constrictive pericarditis may include a thickened pericardium and a septal bounce due to rapid cessation of ventricular filling. The inferior vena cava and hepatic vein may be dilated. Doppler is used to assess diastolic filling. In constrictive pericarditis, the rapid early diastolic filling is reflected in high early inflow velocities with very little contribution from atrial contraction. Doppler may also show respiratory variations in transmitral, transtricuspid, pulmonary, and hepatic flows.

Cardiac catheterization is performed if echocardiography is inconclusive. The prominent $x$ and $y$ descent, dip and plateau in RV diastolic pressure ("square-root" sign), and impaired diastolic filling are seen with right heart catheterization. Catheterization can also show the equalization of the end-diastolic pressures of the heart. CT and MRI are both sensitive means of visualizing the pericardial and aiding in diagnosis [18, 19].

Effusive constrictive pericarditis describes a pericardial effusion, resulting in pericardial tamponade in conjunction with a thickened visceral pericardium causing constriction, and may represent a transition between acute pericarditis with pericardial effusion and pericardial constriction.

## *Therapy*

In general pericardial stripping should be considered for symptomatic constrictive pericarditis. Predictors of adverse outcomes following pericardiectomy include advanced age, renal dysfunction, left ventricular dysfunction, pulmonary hypertension, hyponatremia, and disease due to radiation therapy [20, 21].

# References

1.  Spodick DH. Macrophysiology, microphysiology, and anatomy of the pericardium: a synopsis. Am Heart J. 1992;124(4):1046–51.
2.  Lange RA, Hillis LD. Clinical practice. Acute pericarditis. N Engl J Med. 2004;351(21): 2195–202.
3.  Spodick DH. Diagnostic electrocardiographic sequences in acute pericarditis. Significance of PR segment and PR vector changes. Circulation. 1973;48(3):575–80.
4.  Bruce MA, Spodick DH. Atypical electrocardiogram in acute pericarditis: characteristics and prevalence. J Electrocardiol. 1980;13(1):61–6.
5.  Spodick DH. Acute pericarditis: current concepts and practice. JAMA. 2003;289(9):1150–3.
6.  Imazio M et al. Cardiac troponin I in acute pericarditis. J Am Coll Cardiol. 2003;42(12): 2144–8.
7.  Cheitlin MD et al. ACC/AHA/ASE 2003 guideline update for the clinical application of echocardiography: summary article: a report of the American College of Cardiology/American Heart Association Task Force on Practice Guidelines (ACC/AHA/ASE Committee to Update the 1997 Guidelines for the Clinical Application of Echocardiography). Circulation. 2003;108(9):1146–62.
8.  Maisch B et al. Guidelines on the diagnosis and management of pericardial diseases executive summary; The Task force on the diagnosis and management of pericardial diseases of the European Society of Cardiology. Eur Heart J. 2004;25(7):587–610.
9.  Imazio M et al. Colchicine as first-choice therapy for recurrent pericarditis: results of the CORE (COlchicine for REcurrent pericarditis) trial. Arch Intern Med. 2005;165(17):1987–91.

10. Artom G et al. Pretreatment with corticosteroids attenuates the efficacy of colchicine in preventing recurrent pericarditis: a multi-centre all-case analysis. Eur Heart J. 2005;26(7):723–7.
11. Reddy PS et al. Cardiac tamponade: hemodynamic observations in man. Circulation. 1978;58(2):265–72.
12. Santamore WP et al. Effects of increased pericardial pressure on the coupling between the ventricles. Cardiovasc Res. 1990;24(9):768–76.
13. Spodick DH. Pathophysiology of cardiac tamponade. Chest. 1998;113(5):1372–8.
14. Spodick DH. Acute cardiac tamponade. N Engl J Med. 2003;349(7):684–90.
15. Himelman RB et al. Inferior vena cava plethora with blunted respiratory response: a sensitive echocardiographic sign of cardiac tamponade. J Am Coll Cardiol. 1988;12(6):1470–7.
16. Kronzon I, Cohen ML, Winer HE. Contribution of echocardiography to the understanding of the pathophysiology of cardiac tamponade. J Am Coll Cardiol. 1983;1(4):1180–2.
17. Kronzon I, Cohen ML, Winer HE. Diastolic atrial compression: a sensitive echocardiographic sign of cardiac tamponade. J Am Coll Cardiol. 1983;2(4):770–5.
18. Masui T, Finck S, Higgins CB. Constrictive pericarditis and restrictive cardiomyopathy: evaluation with MR imaging. Radiology. 1992;182(2):369–73.
19. Wang ZJ, et al. CT and MR imaging of pericardial disease. Radiographics. 2003;23 Spec No:S167–80.
20. Bertog SC et al. Constrictive pericarditis: etiology and cause-specific survival after pericardiectomy. J Am Coll Cardiol. 2004;43(8):1445–52.
21. Ling LH et al. Constrictive pericarditis in the modern era: evolving clinical spectrum and impact on outcome after pericardiectomy. Circulation. 1999;100(13):1380–6.

# Chapter 8
# Prevention of Bacterial Endocarditis

Bacterial endocarditis, although uncommon, is a life-threatening disease with substantial morbidity and mortality. Endocarditis usually develops in individuals with underlying structural cardiac defects who develop bacteremia with organisms that have a predilection to invade cardiac structures.

Endocarditis usually occurs after a transient bacteremia seeds either a damaged heart valve or the endocardium near anatomic defects. Although bacteremia is common following a variety of activities in our daily lives as well as in invasive procedures, only certain bacteria commonly cause endocarditis. The risk of endocarditis depends on both the structural cardiac abnormalities and the degree of bacteremia, and so preventive efforts are focused on patients with structural cardiac abnormalities. The individuals at highest risk are those who have prosthetic heart valves, a previous history of endocarditis (even in the absence of other heart disease), complex unrepaired cyanotic congenital heart disease, or surgically constructed systemic pulmonary shunts or conduits [1].

The incidence of endocarditis following most procedures in patients with underlying cardiac disease is low and as such, routine use of antibiotic prophylaxis in all patients with structural heart disease has recently come into question. Over and above this, the data on the efficacy of pre-procedural prophylaxis is also limited, but even if one assumes that prophylaxis is always efficacious, the number needed to treat in order to prevent one event of endocarditis is quite high. Bearing this in mind, professional societies in both the United States and Europe have formulated approaches for endocarditis prophylaxis, weighing the degree to which the patient's underlying condition creates a risk of endocarditis, the risk of bacteremia with the procedure, and the risk-benefit ratio of the prophylactic antimicrobial regimen under consideration [2, 3]. In the United States, the American Heart Association (AHA) guidelines for antibiotic prophylaxis for certain patients undergoing dental procedures, infected skin, skin structures, or musculoskeletal tissue procedures, and respiratory procedures are the most widely followed [2]. Procedures involving the genitourinary tract and the gastrointestinal tract no longer require antibiotic prophylaxis for endocarditis purposes according to the most contemporary guidelines.

S. Hollenberg and S. Heitner, *Cardiology in Family Practice: A Practical Guide*,
Current Clinical Practice 1, DOI 10.1007/978-1-61779-385-1_8,
© Springer Science+Business Media, LLC 2012

While population-based studies have previously classified patients according to their lifetime risk of developing endocarditis according to the comorbidities and degree of structural heart disease [1], the AHA now recommends classifying patients according to the risk of developing an adverse outcome in the event of endocarditis [2]. Antibiotic prophylaxis is currently recommended only for patients at high risk for developing an adverse outcome should they develop endocarditis. Table 8.1 describes the cardiac conditions associated with the highest risk of developing adverse outcomes from endocarditis.

**Table 8.1** Cardiac conditions at highest risk of developing adverse outcomes from infective endocarditis and for which prophylaxis is recommended (Adapted from Wilson et al. [2])

Prosthetic cardiac valves, including bioprosthetic and homograft valves
Previous bacterial endocarditis
Unrepaired cyanotic congenital heart disease including palliative systemic-pulmonary shunt construction (e.g., transposition of the great arteries, tetralogy of Fallot, Fontan, and Rastelli shunts)
Completely repaired congenital heart defect with prosthetic material or device, but only during the first 6 months after the procedure

All patients with conditions listed in Table 8.1 who are undergoing dental procedures that involve manipulation of gingival tissue or the periapical region of teeth or perforation of the oral mucosa should receive pre-procedural prophylaxis. Those patients with planned biopsies or surgical procedures that involve infected skin, skin structures, or musculoskeletal tissue should also receive prophylaxis. Respiratory tract procedures than involve incision of the mucosa (e.g., tonsillectomy or adenoidectomy) should receive prophylaxis. Agents recommended are listed in Table 8.2.

**Table 8.2** Endocarditis prophylactic regimens for dental, oral, respiratory and skin or soft tissue procedures (Adapted from Wilson et al. [2])

| Situation | Agent | Regimen[a] |
|---|---|---|
| Standard general prophylaxis | Amoxicillin | Adults: 2 g; children 50 mg/kg orally 1 h before procedure |
| Unable to take oral medications | Ampicillin | Adults: 2 g IM or IV; Children 50 mg/kg IM or IV within 30 min before procedure |
| Penicillin allergic | Clindamycin or | Adults: 600 mg; children 20 mg/kg orally 1 h before procedure |
| | Cefadroxil[b] or | Adults 2 g; children 50 mg/kg |
| | Cephalexin[b] or | Orally 1 h before procedure |
| | Azithromycin | Adults: 500 mg; children 15 mg/kg orally 1 h before procedure |
| Penicillin allergic and unable to take oral medications | Clindamycin or | Adults: 600 mg; children 20 mg/kg IV within 30 min before procedure |
| | Cefazolin | Adults: 1.0 g; children 25 mg/kg IM or IV 30 min before procedure |

[a] Total pediatric dose should not exceed the adult dose
[b] Cephalosporins should not be used in patients with an immediate-type hypersensitivity reaction (urticaria, angioedema, or anaphylaxis) to penicillins

Of note, a temporal relationship between gastrointestinal and genitourinary procedures and the development of endocarditis has not been conclusively demonstrated, and as such prophylactic antibiotics are no longer routinely recommended.

Antibiotic therapy should be directed at the most common organisms associated with each medical procedure. Alpha-hemolytic *Streptococci* of the *viridans* group is associated with procedures involving the oral and respiratory. The AHA now recommends that only a single pre-procedure antibiotic dose be given for dental, respiratory, and infected skin or soft tissue procedures [2]. The recommended regimen is amoxicillin, 2 g orally pre-procedure, a dose that has prolonged serum levels and inhibitory activity. Erythromycin is no longer recommended for patients with an allergy to penicillin; clindamycin, cephalexin, and cefadroxil or azithromycin should be used [2].

It is important to recognize that when endocarditis develops in individuals with underlying cardiac conditions, the severity of the disease and the ensuing morbidity can be variable. No randomized controlled trials in patients have demonstrated definitely that antibiotic prophlyaxis provides protection against procedure-induced endocarditis. In this area, as in most of medicine, adaptation of general guidelines to individual patients is necessary. Prophylaxis is particularly important for individuals in whom endocardial infection would be associated with high morbidity and mortality.

# References

1. Steckelberg JM, Wilson WR. Risk factors for infective endocarditis. Infect Dis Clin North Am. 1993;7(1):9–19.
2. Wilson W et al. Prevention of infective endocarditis: guidelines from the American Heart Association: a guideline from the American Heart Association Rheumatic Fever, Endocarditis, and Kawasaki Disease Committee, Council on Cardiovascular Disease in the Young, and the Council on Clinical Cardiology, Council on Cardiovascular Surgery and Anesthesia, and the Quality of Care and Outcomes Research Interdisciplinary Working Group. Circulation. 2007; 116(15):1736–54.
3. Horstkotte D et al. Guidelines on prevention, diagnosis and treatment of infective endocarditis executive summary; the task force on infective endocarditis of the European Society of Cardiology. Eur Heart J. 2004;25(3):267–76.

# Chapter 9
# Hyperlipidemia

Cardiovascular disease (CVD) is the leading cause of death in the United States for both men and women. Although the precise number of people with elevated lipids depends on the definition chosen, it is clear that hyperlipidemia is one of the most important modifiable risk factors for coronary heart disease (CHD) in the United States [1].

Lipids are transported in lipoproteins – complex compounds that contain a non-polar core of esterified cholesterol and triglyceride, covered by a polar surface layer that is made up of apolipoproteins, phospholipids, and free cholesterol. The major plasma lipoproteins – chylomicrons, very-low-density-lipoproteins (VLDL), low-density lipoproteins (LDL), and high-density lipoproteins (HDL) are distinguished by lipid content, size, density, electrophoretic mobility, and surface apoproteins. In hyperlipidemia, circulating levels of lipids or lipoproteins are abnormal because of genetic and environmental conditions that alter the production, breakdown, or clearance of plasma lipoproteins from the circulation.

The National Cholesterol Education Program Adult Treatment Panel (NCEP ATP) issues guidelines for the detection, evaluation, and treatment of high blood cholesterol in adults. The latest version published in 2004 (NCEP ATP III) focused on more aggressive treatment, better identification of patients at risk of developing coronary artery disease, defining new levels at which low HDL becomes a major heart disease risk factor, therapeutic lifestyle changes to prevent coronary artery disease, greater awareness of the metabolic syndrome, and increased attention on the treatment of high triglycerides [1]. NCEP ATP II focused on intensifying lipid-lowering therapy in patients with established CHD. While the NCEP ATP III affirms the importance of such efforts, it underscores primary prevention in patients at sufficiently high risk of developing atherosclerotic disease according to their 10-year Framingham risk. The ATP III approach discusses screening for hyperlipidemia, and then calibrates the intensity of lipid-lowering efforts to the degree of cardiovascular risk (see Fig. 9.1).

S. Hollenberg and S. Heitner, *Cardiology in Family Practice: A Practical Guide*, 141
Current Clinical Practice 1, DOI 10.1007/978-1-61779-385-1_9,
© Springer Science+Business Media, LLC 2012

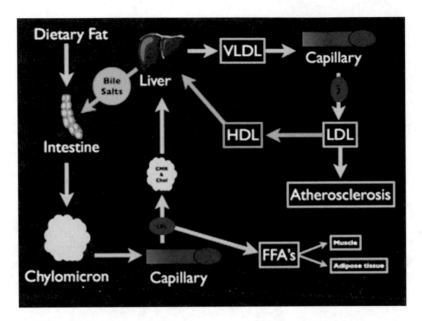

**Fig. 9.1** Outline of lipoprotein metabolism

## Screening

The NCEP ATP III recommends screening every 5 years for all adults over the age of 20 [1]. A fasting lipid profile should contain total cholesterol, LDL, HDL, and triglycerides. If any of these values are abnormal, before initiating drug therapy the recommendation is that patients be screened for secondary causes of dyslipidemia. These secondary causes include diabetes, hypothyroidism, obstructive liver disease, chronic kidney disease, and drugs that might affect the total cholesterol, LDL, and HDL levels (see Table **9.1**).

**Table 9.1** Classification of LDL, HDL, and total cholesterol

| LDL | | Total cholesterol | | HDL | | Triglycerides | |
|---|---|---|---|---|---|---|---|
| <70 | Goal in very high risk | <200 | Desirable | <40 | Low | <150 | Normal |
| <100 | Optimal | 200–239 | Borderline High | >40 | High | 150=199 | Borderline |
| 100–129 | Near Borderline | >240 | High | | | 200–499 | High |
| 130–159 | Borderline High | | | | | >500 | Very high |
| 160–180 | High | | | | | | |
| >190 | Very High | | | | | | |

Adapted from Expert Panel on Detection Evaluation and Treatment of High Blood Cholesterol in Adults [1]; Grundy et al. [5]

# Risk Categories

A key principle underpinning the ATP III guidelines is that the intensity of lipid-lowering therapy should be adjusted to the individual's absolute risk for CHD. Both the short-term (≤10 year) and long-term (>10 year) risk should be taken into consideration. Risk assessment is carried out according to the Framingham risk score, which is derived from observational data over the long-term (Tables 9.2 and 9.3). The risk factors included in the Framingham calculation are: age, total cholesterol, HDL cholesterol, systolic blood pressure, treatment for hypertension, and cigarette smoking [2].

## *Very High Risk*

On the basis of more recent data from the Heart Protection Study and the PROVE-IT trial, this newer risk category was added to the NCEP ATP III classification. These patients are defined as having established CVD plus either multiple major risk factors (especially diabetes), severe and poorly controlled risk factors (especially continued cigarette smoking), the metabolic syndrome (especially high triglycerides >200 mg/dL plus non-HDL-C 130 mg/dL with low HDL-C <40 mg/dL), or presentation with acute coronary syndromes.

## *High Risk*

The criteria for high risk include patients with CHD or CHD risk equivalents. Risk equivalents carry the same risk as coronary artery disease and include diabetes mellitus, peripheral vascular disease, carotid artery disease, abdominal aortic aneurysm, and a calculated 10-year risk of a coronary event >20% by the Framingham risk score (Tables 9.2 and 9.3).

## *Moderately High risk*

Patients are categorized as moderately high risk if they have two or more risk factors and a 10-year risk for a coronary event between 10–20% based on the Framingham risk score (Tables 9.2 and 9.3).

## *Moderate Risk*

Patients are considered at moderate risk if they have two or more risk factors and a 10-year risk for a coronary event of <10% based on the Framingham risk score (Tables 9.2 and 9.3).

**Table 9.2** Estimate of 10-year risk for men and women

| Age | Points | |
|---|---|---|
| | Men | Women |
| 20–34 | −9 | −7 |
| 35–39 | −4 | −3 |
| 40–44 | 0 | 0 |
| 45–49 | 3 | 3 |
| 50–54 | 6 | 6 |
| 55–59 | 8 | 8 |
| 60–69 | 10 | 10 |
| 65–69 | 11 | 12 |
| 70–74 | 12 | 14 |
| 75–79 | 13 | 16 |

| | Age 20–39 | | Age 40–49 | | Age 50–59 | | Age 60–69 | | Age 70–79 | |
|---|---|---|---|---|---|---|---|---|---|---|
| | M | W | M | W | M | W | M | W | M | W |
| *Total cholesterol* | | | | | | | | | | |
| <160 | 0 | 0 | 0 | 0 | 0 | 0 | 0 | 0 | 0 | 0 |
| 160–199 | 4 | 4 | 3 | 3 | 2 | 2 | 1 | 1 | 0 | 1 |
| 200–239 | 7 | 8 | 5 | 6 | 3 | 4 | 1 | 2 | 0 | 1 |
| 240–279 | 9 | 11 | 6 | 8 | 4 | 5 | 2 | 3 | 1 | 2 |
| >280 | 11 | 13 | 8 | 10 | 5 | 7 | 3 | 4 | 1 | 2 |
| *Smoking* | | | | | | | | | | |
| Nonsmoker | 0 | 0 | 0 | 0 | 0 | 0 | 0 | 0 | 0 | 0 |
| Smoker | 8 | 9 | 5 | 7 | 3 | 4 | 1 | 2 | 1 | 1 |

| HDL | Points (men and women) |
|---|---|
| >60 | −1 |
| 50–59 | 0 |
| 40–49 | 1 |
| <40 | 2 |

| Systolic BP | Untreated | | Treated | |
|---|---|---|---|---|
| | M | W | M | W |
| <120 | 0 | 0 | 0 | 0 |
| 120–129 | 0 | 1 | 1 | 3 |
| 130–139 | 1 | 2 | 2 | 4 |
| 140–159 | 1 | 3 | 2 | 5 |
| >160 | 2 | 4 | 3 | 6 |

Adapted from the Expert Panel on Detection, Evaluation, and Treatment of High Blood Cholesterol in Adults [1]

**Table 9.3** Calculation of a patient's 10-year risk

| Total points | 10-Year risk (%) | |
| --- | --- | --- |
| | M | W |
| <0 | <1 | <1 |
| 0–4 | 1 | <1 |
| 5–6 | 2 | <1 |
| 7 | 3 | <1 |
| 8 | 4 | <1 |
| 9 | 5 | 1 |
| 10 | 6 | 1 |
| 11 | 8 | 1 |
| 12 | 0 | 1 |
| 13 | 12 | 2 |
| 14 | 16 | 2 |
| 15 | 0 | 3 |
| 16 | 25 | 4 |
| 17 | 30 | 5 |
| 18 | >30 | 6 |
| 19 | >30 | 8 |
| 20 | >30 | 11 |
| 21 | >30 | 14 |
| 22 | >30 | 17 |
| 23 | >30 | 22 |
| 24 | >30 | 27 |
| >25 | >30 | >30 |

Adapted from the Expert Panel on Detection, Evaluation, and Treatment of High Blood Cholesterol in Adults [1]

## *Low Risk*

Patients with zero or one risk factor or with a 10-year risk of <10% according to the Framingham risk score.

An online Framingham risk calculator is available through the National Heart Lung and Blood Institute at the following web address: http://hp2010.nhlbihin.net/atpiii/calculator.asp?usertype=prof.

## *Risk Factors*

Risk factors include smoking, hypertension (blood pressure >140/90 mmHg or on antihypertensive medications), low HDL (<40 mg/dL), first-degree relatives with premature CHD (in males, age <55; in females, age <65), age (men >45 years old; women >55 years old). Hypertriglyceridemia is also an independent risk factor for CHD, but it is not included in the Framingham calculation [3]. An HDL cholesterol of >60 mg/dL is considered protective, and one risk factor should be removed from the total score [1].

## Metabolic Syndrome

Metabolic syndrome is a constellation of features that ultimately greatly increase a person's risk of developing diabetes mellitus and CVD (almost double the risk) [4]. Three of the following criteria are required to make the diagnosis of metabolic syndrome: (1) abdominal obesity (waist circumference of >35 in. in women or >40 in. in men), (2) elevated triglyceride level (>150 mg/dL), (3) a low HDL level (<40 mg/dL in men or <50 mg/dL in women), (4) high fasting glucose level (>110 mg/dL), and (5) high blood pressure (>130/85 mmHg).

## *Therapy*

Therapeutic lifestyle changes should be initiated for all patients with an LDL that is above goal. Recommended lifestyle changes include reduction in saturated fat (to <7% of total calories), cholesterol intake (to <200 mg/day), weight reduction, and increased physical activity. Patients in the high or moderately high-risk categories should be encouraged to change lifestyle regardless of their LDL levels. Lifestyle-related risk factors include obesity, elevated triglycerides, low HDL, metabolic syndrome or physical inactivity.

It is reasonable to aim for a goal LDL <70 mg/dL in very-high-risk patients [5]. For patients at high risk, the recommended goal LDL is <100 mg/dL. In the high-risk population in whom LDL remains >100 mg/dL despite lifestyle changes, a lipid-lowering drug should also be initiated. A second therapeutic goal, particularly when the starting LDL is not especially high, is aiming for a 30–40% reduction after drug and lifestyle intervention [1]. If a high-risk patient has elevated triglycerides or low HDL, then additional pharmacotherapy with either a fibrate or nicotinic acid can be considered. Importantly, the clinician should keep in mind that there might be a higher incidence of adverse drug reactions when combination therapy is employed.

For patients at moderately high risk, the goal LDL is <130 mg/dL. Lifestyle changes should be initiated, and lipid lowering medications should be started if the LDL is >160 mg/dL. A therapeutic option is to lower the LDL to <100 mg/dL, and to initiate drug therapy in those patients with a baseline LDL of 100–129 mg/dL in whom lifestyle changes have failed [5]. As with high-risk patients, a reduction of 30–40% is recommended [5].

For patients at low risk, the goal LDL is <160 mg/dL. Lifestyle changes should be initiated. Drug therapy is optional and is initiated only if the LDL cholesterol is between 160 and 189 mg/dL after adequate lifestyle changes. If the LDL is >190 mg/dL, then drug therapy should be initiated.

Elevated triglycerides can occur in patients with obesity, diabetes, hypothyroidism, nephrotic syndrome, estrogen replacement therapy, or immunosuppressive therapy, and other familial genetic disorders. Achievement of the LDL goal is particularly important for patients with a triglyceride level >150 mg/dL. Weight loss and increased physical activity should be emphasized. The importance of triglycerides has been stressed in ATP III with the introduction of non-HDL (total cholesterol − HDL cholesterol) as a therapeutic target. These targets are 30 mg/dL higher than the corresponding LDL targets, thus recommending therapy at lower LDL levels when triglycerides exceed 150 (recall that total cholesterol = TG/5 + HDL + LDL). In patients with very high triglycerides a low fat diet, weight loss, increased physical activity, and a triglyceride lowering drug should be initiated. Potential pharmacotherapy includes nicotinic acid, fibrates, or omega-3 fatty acids [1].

Metabolic syndrome is a risk factor for developing CVD as well as type-2 diabetes mellitus. Lifestyle modification (weight reduction, increased physical activity, and diet) and cardiovascular risk reduction (lipid lowering, blood pressure and tight glycemic control) are crucial preventive measures for these patients.

Subsequent to the publication of the NCEP ATP III guidelines in 2001, an update was released in 2004, the purpose of which was to incorporate important data that had become available since the initial publication.

The Heart Prevention Study (HPS), a primary prevention study, showed a reduction in all-cause mortality, major vascular events, and coronary events in high-risk patients despite the level of LDL when using simvastatin as compared to placebo [6]. The treatment group had reductions in all-cause mortality (13%), major vascular events (24%), coronary death (18%), nonfatal MI or coronary death (27%), fatal or nonfatal stroke (25%), and coronary revascularization (24%) [6]. A subgroup analysis showed similar reductions in risk regardless of LDL levels.

Along similar lines, the JUPITER study tested the effect of statins in 17,802 apparently healthy low-risk patients with normal LDL levels (<130 mg/dL) but elevated high-sensitivity C-reactive protein (hsCRP) levels. In this population, patients treated with 20 mg of rosuvastatin had a 50% reduction in LDL and 37% reduction in hsCRP, and showed a significant 44% reduction in the combined endpoint (death, stroke, myocardial infarction, hospital admission for acute coronary syndromes, and arterial revascularization) when compared to placebo [7]. Significant reductions in the individual endpoints were seen as well, although the absolute risk reductions were modest (for the primary endpoint, 0.77 vs. 1.36 events per 100 person-years, with lower absolute reductions for the components) [7]. This trial showed that even in these healthy low risk patients, elevated hsCRP levels were an independent marker for CVD risk.

The Prospective Study of Pravastatin in the Elderly at Risk (PROSPER) study showed a similar benefit to statin use in high-risk elderly patients, a cohort that had previously been excluded from the older major clinical trials [8].

A substudy of the Antihypertension and Lipid-Lowering Treatment to Prevent Heart Attack Trial-Lipid-Lowering Trial (ALLHAT-LLT), showed that the benefits of statin therapy extended to women and minority groups, something that might have been predicted but had not been demonstrated unequivocally in a randomized trial [9].

The Anglo-Scandinavian Cardiac Outcomes Trial (ASCOT) underscored the utility of statins as primary prevention in the at-risk population with hypertension, and relatively low total cholesterol levels, regardless of age [10].

Which LDL goal to target was tested in the Pravastatin or Atorvastatin Evaluation and Infection Therapy – Thrombolysis in Myocardial Infarction 22 Trial (PROVE-IT TIMI-22) study [11]. This study randomized 4,162 patients with acute coronary syndromes (mean LDL of 106 mg/dL) to 40 mg of pravastatin (which decreased LDL to 95 mg/dL) or 80 mg of atorvastatin (which decreased LDL to 62 mg/dL). The greater decrease with atorvastatin was associated with a significant (16% relative and a 3.9% absolute) reduction in the combined end point of death, MI, stroke, rehospitalization for ischemia, and revascularization. This was the first large-scale study to show an added clinical benefit in more intensive LDL lowering (below 100 mg/dL) in post-ACS patients, and that perhaps a goal of <70 mg/dL is more appropriate in these patients. In a post-hoc analysis of this study, it was noted that patients with a low hsCRP (<2.0 mg/L) levels after statin therapy tended to have better clinical outcomes when compared to those with higher hsCRP levels, regardless of the resultant level of LDL cholesterol [12]. It has also been demonstrated that if statin therapy is initiated in the in-patient setting, there is a higher likelihood of medication adherence [13]. Furthermore, intensification of statin therapy in patients with stable CVD to drive the LDL levels to <100 mg/dL has also shown an incremental benefit [14].

It would seem that while the evidence underpinning the current NCEP ATP III guidelines is robust, the goals recommended may in fact be too lax, and an update will almost certainly include aiming at an LDL <70 mg/dL in certain populations, and measuring hsCRP in others.

## Lipid-Lowering Drugs

Table 9.4 lists the lipid-lowering agents and expected changes in the lipid profile. HMG-CoA inhibitors, or statins, inhibit the rate-limiting step in cholesterol

**Table 9.4** Drugs affecting lipoprotein metabolism

| Drug class | Lipid/Lipoprotein | Effects |
| --- | --- | --- |
| HMG CoA reductase inhibitors (statins) | LDL | Decrease by 18–55% |
| | HDL | Increase by 5–15% |
| | TG | Decrease by 7–30% |
| Bile acid sequestrants | LDL | Decrease by 15–30% |
| | HDL | Increase by 3–5% |
| | TG | No change or increase |
| Nicotinic acid | LDL | Decrease by 5–25% |
| | HDL | Increase by 15–35% |
| | TG | Decrease by 20–50% |
| Fibric acids | LDL | Decrease by 5–20% (may be increased in patients with high TG) |
| | HDL | Increase by 10–20% |
| | TG | Decrease by 20–50% |

Adapted from the Expert Panel on Detection, Evaluation, and Treatment of High Blood Cholesterol in Adults [1]

biosynthesis. Statins are the first-line agents for all patients with mixed dyslipidemia. The potency of the individual statins for LDL reduction differs, with rosuvastatin being the most potent, and lovastatin being the least potent of the agents. The most frequent side effects are a mild increase in liver enzymes and myalgias. Only 1% of patients taking statins will experience hepatotoxicity with liver enzymes increasing more than three-fold the upper limit of normal. This is most frequently seen within the first 3 months of starting therapy, and is usually subclinical and transient. Rare patients will have continued significant elevation, develop the symptoms of hepatitis and require discontinuation of the statin. The hepatotoxicity is reversible after the offending agent is discontinued. Myalgias are equally infrequent, also occurring in <1% patients, but the risk of myopathy is increased with concomitant use of fibrates, nicotinic acid, erythromycin, and cyclosporin. Very rarely patients may exhibit evidence of myositis (myopathy in the setting of inflammatory changes in the muscles associated with fever and elevated serum muscle enzymes) or even rhabdomyolysis. Decreasing the dose or changing from one statin to another is sometimes helpful in dealing with myalgias, but some patients may not be able to tolerate the symptoms and the statin may need to be discontinued.

Fibric acid derivatives (fibrates) increase fatty acid oxidation and lipoprotein lipase activity, resulting in lower triglyceride levels and higher HDL levels. Fibrates are generally well tolerated. Side effects from fibrates include cholelithiasis, gastrointestinal upset, and myopathies (more frequent with concomitant statins).

Nicotinic acid (niacin) inhibits the mobilization of free fatty acids from peripheral tissues to the liver, decreasing hepatic VLDL synthesis and release. Niacin is the most effective agent available for raising HDL levels. Side effects with nicotinic acid are common but usually mild and tolerance develops with time. The most frequently reported side effects include flushing, nausea, itching, paresthesias, insulin resistance, and hyperuricemia. Pretreatment with aspirin 30 min prior to ingestion often helps reduce flushing. Hepatotoxicity is the most serious adverse effect, and liver functions should be monitored.

Bile acid sequestrants interrupt enterohepatic circulation of bile acids, which increases the conversion of endogenous cholesterol to bile acids in an effort to replace their loss in the gastrointestinal tract. Bile acid sequestrants, either alone or in combination with statins can reduce LDL levels. Side effects of these drugs include nausea, bloating, cramping, increased liver enzymes, and decreased absorption of drugs such as digoxin, warfarin, and the fat-soluble vitamins (A, D, E, and K). Bile acid sequestrants can increase triglyceride levels and are therefore not recommended for use as monotherapy.

Ezetimibe is a newer cholesterol-lowering agent that blocks the absorption of cholesterol by the small intestine. Ezetimibe can lower cholesterol when used alone, but is most effective when used in combination with statins. The combination of low doses of ezetimibe and statins can be as effective in lowering LDL as high doses of statins alone [15]. Ezetimibe is generally well tolerated and has little interaction with other medications. The ENHANCE (Ezetimibe and Simvastatin in Hypercholesterolemia Enhances Atherosclerosis Regression) looked at whether the addition of ezetimibe to simvastatin would result in plaque regression via carotid artery ultrasound [16]. This was a randomized, double-blind, 2 year follow-up study on

720 patients with familial hypercholesterolemia, and although clinical end-points were not the focus, there was no demonstrable benefit by the addition of ezetimibe. These results have tempered the early enthusiasm for the use of this novel agent [15, 16] especially in the setting of a possible association with an increase in cancer incidence [17]. Although the issue of carcinogenesis seems to have been resolved [18], there is a lack of compelling evidence to use this agent as first-line therapy. Should the LDL levels remain problematically high despite maximal therapy with other drugs, or in the event that a patient cannot tolerate a statin, it seems reasonable to use ezetimibe.

An excess of dietary saturated fat is associated with an increase in the risk for CVD. Substituting 10% of calories from saturated fatty acid with omega-6 polyunsaturated fatty acid (PUFA) is associated with an 18 mg/dL decrease in LDL. A recent meta-analysis of six trials indicated that replacing saturated fatty acids with PUFA results in lowering of the risk for CVD events by 24% [19]. There are few reported side effects with omega-6 fatty acid therapy, and it is therefore reasonable to use this as additional pharmacotherapy in patients who meet criteria for lipid-lowering therapy.

# References

1. Expert Panel on Detection Evaluation and Treatment of High Blood Cholesterol in Adults. Executive summary of the third report of the National Cholesterol Education Program (NCEP) expert panel on detection, evaluation, and treatment of high blood cholesterol in adults (Adult Treatment Panel III). JAMA. 2001;285:2486–96.
2. Wilson PW et al. Prediction of coronary heart disease using risk factor categories. Circulation. 1998;97(18):1837–47.
3. Austin MA, Hokanson JE, Edwards KL. Hypertriglyceridemia as a cardiovascular risk factor. Am J Cardiol. 1998;81(4A):7B–12.
4. Galassi A, Reynolds K, He J. Metabolic syndrome and risk of cardiovascular disease: a meta-analysis. Am J Med. 2006;119(10):812–9.
5. Grundy SM et al. Implications of recent clinical trials for the National Cholesterol Education Program Adult Treatment Panel III Guidelines. J Am Coll Cardiol. 2004;44(3):720–32.
6. Heart Protection Study Collaborative Group. MRC/BHF Heart Protection Study of cholesterol lowering with simvastatin in 20,536 high-risk individuals: a randomised placebo-controlled trial. Lancet. 2002;360(9326):7–22.
7. Ridker PM et al. Rosuvastatin to prevent vascular events in men and women with elevated C-reactive protein. N Engl J Med. 2008;359(21):2195–207.
8. Shepherd J et al. Pravastatin in elderly individuals at risk of vascular disease (PROSPER): a randomised controlled trial. Lancet. 2002;360(9346):1623–30.
9. ALLHAT Investigators. Major outcomes in moderately hypercholesterolemic, hypertensive patients randomized to pravastatin vs usual care: The Antihypertensive and Lipid-Lowering Treatment to Prevent Heart Attack Trial (ALLHAT-LLT). JAMA. 2002;288(23):2998–3007.
10. Sever PS et al. Prevention of coronary and stroke events with atorvastatin in hypertensive patients who have average or lower-than-average cholesterol concentrations, in the Anglo-Scandinavian Cardiac Outcomes Trial-Lipid Lowering Arm (ASCOT-LLA): a multicentre randomised controlled trial. Lancet. 2003;361(9364):1149–58.
11. Cannon CP et al. Intensive versus moderate lipid lowering with statins after acute coronary syndromes. N Engl J Med. 2004;350:1495–504.

12. Ridker PM et al. C-reactive protein levels and outcomes after statin therapy. N Engl J Med. 2005;352(1):20–8.
13. Fonarow GC et al. Improved treatment of coronary heart disease by implementation of a Cardiac Hospitalization Atherosclerosis Management Program (CHAMP). Am J Cardiol. 2001;87(7):819–22.
14. LaRosa JC et al. Intensive lipid lowering with atorvastatin in patients with stable coronary disease. N Engl J Med. 2005;352(14):1425–35.
15. Davidson MH et al. Ezetimibe coadministered with simvastatin in patients with primary hypercholesterolemia. J Am Coll Cardiol. 2002;40(12):2125–34.
16. Kastelein JJ et al. Simvastatin with or without ezetimibe in familial hypercholesterolemia. N Engl J Med. 2008;358(14):1431–43.
17. Rossebo AB et al. Intensive lipid lowering with simvastatin and ezetimibe in aortic stenosis. N Engl J Med. 2008;359(13):1343–56.
18. Peto R et al. Analyses of cancer data from three ezetimibe trials. N Engl J Med. 2008; 359(13):1357–66.
19. Harris WS et al. Omega-6 fatty acids and risk for cardiovascular disease: a science advisory from the American Heart Association Nutrition Subcommittee of the Council on Nutrition, Physical Activity, and Metabolism; Council on Cardiovascular Nursing; and Council on Epidemiology and Prevention. Circulation. 2009;119(6):902–7.

# Index

S. Hollenberg and S. Heitner, *Cardiology in Family Practice: A Practical Guide*,
Current Clinical Practice 1, DOI 10.1007/978-1-61779-385-1,
© Springer Science+Business Media, LLC 2012